LOW-FAT
WAYS TO
LOSE WEIGHT

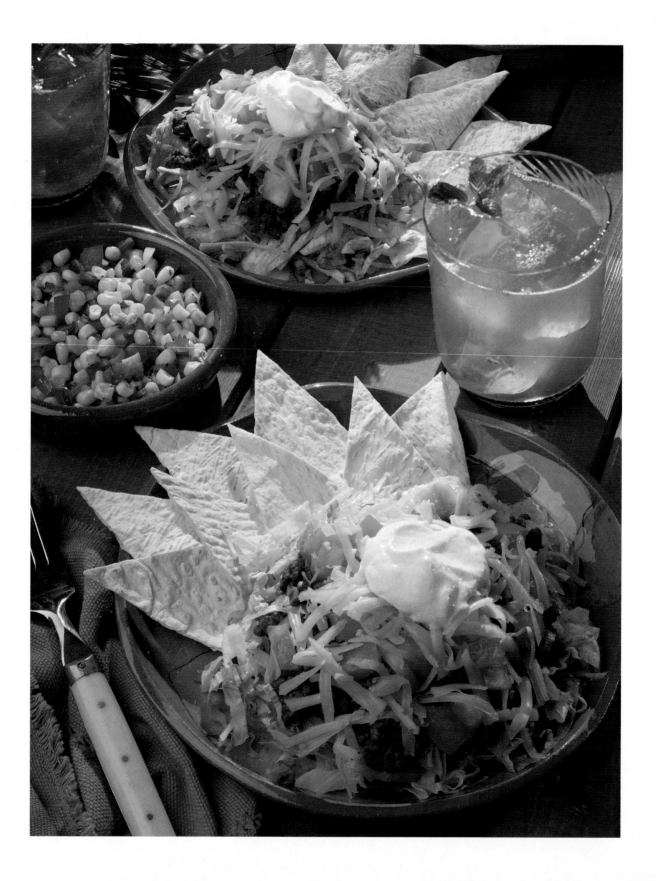

LOW-FAT
WAYS TO
LOSE WEIGHT

COMPILED AND EDITED BY
SUSAN M. MCINTOSH, M.S., R.D.

Oxmoor
House®

Library of Congress Catalog Number: 96-68032   .
ISBN: 0-8487-2208-6
Manufactured in the United States of America
First Printing 1996

Editor-in-Chief: Nancy Fitzpatrick Wyatt
Editorial Director, Special Interest Publications: Ann H. Harvey
Senior Foods Editor: Katherine M. Eakin
Senior Editor, Editorial Services: Olivia Kindig Wells
Art Director: James Boone

LOW-FAT WAYS TO LOSE WEIGHT

Menu and Recipe Consultant: Susan McEwen McIntosh, M.S., R.D.
Assistant Editor: Kelly Hooper Troiano
Assistant Foods Editor: Caroline A. Grant, M.S., R.D.
Copy Editor: Shari K. Wimberly
Editorial Assistant: Kaye Howard Smith
Indexer: Mary Ann Laurens
Assistant Art Director: Cynthia R. Cooper
Designer: Carol Damsky
Senior Photographer: Jim Bathie
Photographers: Howard L. Puckett, *Cooking Light* magazine;
  Ralph Anderson
Senior Photo Stylist: Kay E. Clarke
Photo Stylists: Cindy Manning Barr, *Cooking Light* magazine;
  Virginia R. Cravens
Production and Distribution Director: Phillip Lee
Associate Production Managers: Theresa L. Beste, Vanessa D. Cobbs
Production Coordinator: Marianne Jordan Wilson
Production Assistant: Valerie Heard

Our appreciation to the staff of *Cooking Light* magazine and to the Southern
Progress Corporation library staff for their contributions to this book.

Cover: *Pork Madeira and Mashed Potatoes (menu on page 102)*
Frontispiece: *Taco Salad for Two and Mexican Corn (menu on page 48)*

CONTENTS

LEAN FOR LIFE

*P*ut away the magic milk shakes, diet pills, and high-protein meal plans. Although these may help you lose a few quick pounds, the excess weight can slowly creep back. So what is the answer to losing weight *and* keeping it off? Not suprisingly, it is a diet low in fat and calories! So start your program now with these basic, great-tasting recipes and menus that you can enjoy for a lifetime.

If you've suddenly gone from a size 10 to a size 12, or if you look in the mirror and see bulges that weren't there last year, you probably need to lose a few pounds. You may not think you've gained weight, but the doctor's scales say otherwise.

Most likely you probably know the problems that plague those who are overweight—heart disease, high blood pressure, stroke, diabetes, arthritis, and breathing difficulties. But just what is a healthy weight?

People of the same height can fall within a fairly wide range of weights and be considered healthy. That's because individuals have different amounts of muscle and bone. The chart at the right shows healthy weight ranges for adult men and women of all ages.

The higher your weight is above the healthy range, the greater your risk of having or developing one or more of the problems associated with being overweight.

The location and percentage of weight that's stored as fat also play important roles in health. If you are overweight, consider where the fat is located. Extra pounds around the waist or midsection are linked to a higher risk of heart disease and diabetes. Pudgy thighs, however, don't appear to be detrimental to health.

Weights falling below the healthy range may be caused by underlying health problems, such as anorexia nervosa or appetite loss associated with

other diseases. If you experience a sudden, unintentional loss of weight, it is wise to consult a physician.

ARE YOU OVERWEIGHT?

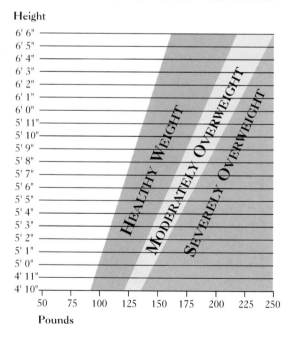

Reference: *Nutrition and Your Health: Dietary Guidelines for Americans,* Fourth Edition, U.S. Department of Agriculture, U.S. Department of Health and Human Services.

WHAT'S THE ANSWER?

So where do you begin once you determine that you are ready to make some permanent lifestyle changes? First, realize that there are two ways to lose weight:

• Eat fewer calories than your body needs for energy.

• Burn extra calories by increasing your level of activity.

To lose 1 pound a week, cut back or burn 500 calories per day (3,500 calories equal 1 pound). You could burn about 200 calories a day by simply walking briskly 30 to 40 minutes. Combine walking with some cutbacks in fat and calories, and the result should be gradual weight loss.

Avoid diets of fewer than 1,200 calories a day unless recommended by your doctor. Severely limiting your food intake can prevent you from getting the nutrients you need to stay healthy.

Don't try to lose weight too quickly—the slower you take off extra pounds, the greater the chance that they will stay off. The newest recommendations set a reasonable pace for weight loss at ½ to 1 pound per week.

If your weight is over the healthy range, realize that you'll benefit even if you lose only a few pounds. Try to avoid "yo-yo dieting." It's healthier to maintain a steady weight, even if it's a bit above normal, than to repeatedly lose and regain.

Calorie Countdown

All foods contain calories—some more than others. The number of calories a food contains depends on the amounts of fat, protein, carbohydrate, and alcohol present in the food. Fat contains 9 calories per gram, protein and carbohydrate each contain 4 calories per gram, and alcohol contains 7 calories per gram.

Because fat provides so many calories per gram, foods high in fat are also high in calories. But even if a food is low-fat, its calories still count and can contribute to weight gain.

Recent dietary guidelines provide practical advice on what Americans should eat to stay healthy:

• Eat a variety of foods.

• Balance the food you eat with physical activity to maintain or improve your weight.

• Choose a diet with plenty of grain products, vegetables, and fruit.

• Choose a diet low in fat, saturated fat, and cholesterol.

• Choose a diet moderate in sugars.

• Choose a diet moderate in salt and sodium.

• If you drink alcoholic beverages, do so in moderation.

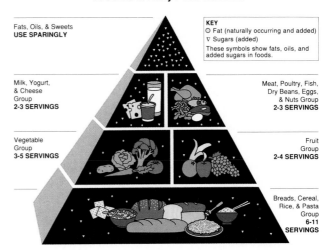

Food Guide Pyramid
A Guide to Daily Food Choices

Fats, Oils, & Sweets
USE SPARINGLY

KEY
○ Fat (naturally occurring and added)
▽ Sugars (added)
These symbols show fats, oils, and added sugars in foods.

Milk, Yogurt, & Cheese Group
2-3 SERVINGS

Meat, Poultry, Fish, Dry Beans, Eggs, & Nuts Group
2-3 SERVINGS

Vegetable Group
3-5 SERVINGS

Fruit Group
2-4 SERVINGS

Breads, Cereal, Rice, & Pasta Group
6-11 SERVINGS

Reference: *Nutrition and Your Health: Dietary Guidelines for Americans*, Fourth Edition, U.S. Department of Agriculture, U.S. Department of Health and Human Services.

The Food Guide Pyramid is a visual representation of the dietary guidelines. Most of the food that you eat should come from groups at the base of the pyramid—breads, cereal, rice, pasta, vegetables, and fruit. These foods, rich in vitamins, minerals, complex carbohydrates, and dietary fiber, contribute to overall health and may help prevent heart disease, cancer, and other diseases.

The pyramid also shows that fats and sweets should be limited. Although fats and sugars are obvious in butter and candy, they're also present in other foods. This is illustrated by circles (symbolizing fat) and triangles (symbolizing sugar) throughout the pyramid.

SUPERMARKET SAVVY

The first step to preparing low-fat, low-calorie meals is to buy the right ingredients at the supermarket. Grains, pasta, vegetables, and fruit are naturally low in fat and are excellent sources of complex carbohydrates, fiber, vitamins, and minerals. Careful reading of labels on convenience products will allow you to choose from a variety of low- and reduced-fat items that are widely available.

By limiting butter, fatty meats, and high-fat dairy products, you will automatically restrict your saturated fat and cholesterol intake. High levels of saturated fat and cholesterol in diets have been linked to a greater risk of heart disease.

Use the table below to guide you as you stock your pantry and refrigerator with ingredients that are low in fat and calories.

HEALTHY INGREDIENT SUBSTITUTIONS

Recipe calls for:	Use:
FATS AND OILS	
Butter or margarine	Reduced-calorie margarine or margarine with 2 grams or less saturated fat per tablespoon
Mayonnaise	Nonfat or reduced-fat mayonnaise
Oil or shortening	Canola, corn, olive, peanut, safflower, soybean, sunflower, or other oil high in monounsaturated or polyunsaturated fat
Salad dressing	Nonfat or oil-free salad dressing
DAIRY PRODUCTS	
American, Cheddar, colby, Monterey Jack, mozzarella, and Swiss cheeses	Reduced-fat cheeses with 5 grams or less fat per ounce
Cottage cheese	Nonfat or 1% low-fat cottage cheese
Cream cheese	Nonfat or light cream cheese, Neufchâtel cheese
Ricotta cheese	Nonfat or light ricotta cheese
Ice cream	Nonfat or low-fat ice cream, nonfat or low-fat frozen yogurt, sherbet
Milk, whole or 2%	Skim milk, ½% milk, or 1% milk
Milk, evaporated	Evaporated skimmed milk
Sour cream	Nonfat or low-fat sour cream, nonfat or low-fat yogurt
Whipping cream	Evaporated skimmed milk
MEATS, POULTRY, FISH, AND EGGS	
Bacon	Canadian bacon, turkey bacon, lean ham
High-fat cuts of beef, veal, lamb, and pork	Chicken or turkey breast, lean cuts of meat trimmed of all visible fat
Ground beef	Ground round, extra-lean ground beef, ground turkey breast
Luncheon meat	Sliced, cooked turkey or chicken breast, lean ham or roast beef
Poultry	Skinned poultry
Tuna packed in oil	Tuna packed in water
Egg, whole	2 egg whites or ¼ cup frozen egg substitute, thawed

TAKE-IT-OFF TIPS

Cooking methods and ingredients added during preparation can turn lean foods into high-fat foods. Here are some techniques to remember.

• Avoid deep-fat frying meats, chicken, fish, and vegetables, and remember that overcooking vegetables destroys vitamins and minerals. Use one of the following low-fat cooking methods instead: broiling, grilling, poaching, roasting, sautéing, steaming, or stir-frying.

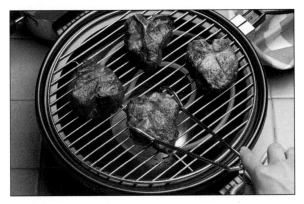

Grilling

• Trim all visible fat from meat and poultry before cooking. Remove the skin from poultry before or after cooking.

• Remove or omit oil from marinades for meats, fish, and poultry by substituting water or broth.

• Decrease the fat in cooking by eliminating added fat (such as cooking oil or butter), decreasing the amount called for in a recipe, and sautéing in

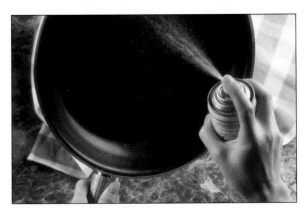

Using vegetable cooking spray

nonstick skillets or regular skillets coated with vegetable cooking spray.

• Microwave vegetables, fruit, fish, poultry, and some meats to preserve flavor, texture, color, and nutrients with little or no added fat.

• Broil and roast meats, poultry, and fish on a rack in a broiler pan to allow fat to drip away.

• Cook tough cuts of meat slowly by braising or stewing. Be sure to remove fat from the drippings as described below.

• Use a fat skimmer or fat-separating cup to remove fat from meat drippings or soup stock. Or chill the meat drippings, and skim off any hardened fat.

• Spoon cooked ground meat into a colander to drain excess fat. To further reduce the fat content of cooked meat, pat it with paper towels after draining. If other ingredients are to be added back to the skillet, wipe drippings from skillet with a paper towel.

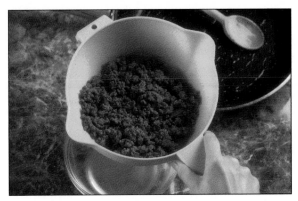

Draining

• Season grains, legumes, and pasta with herbs instead of high-fat ingredients, such as gravy, butter, or a cream sauce, that can turn healthy foods into calorie- and fat-laden ones.

• Cook with wines and other spirits to add flavor but not fat. Most of the alcohol and calories will evaporate during cooking, leaving only the flavor behind. Small amounts of extracts, such as vanilla and almond, also add flavor without adding fat.

• Remember that portion sizes are important in healthy cooking. Food scales and measuring cups can assist you in determining proper portion sizes as well as correct ingredient amounts.

Low-Fat Menu Plans

According to major health advisory groups, an ideal diet derives 30 percent or fewer of its calories from fat, at least 50 percent from carbohydrates, and about 20 percent from protein.

Sound confusing? Before you run for your calculator to plan supper, take a look at the following menus. All meet the above guidelines for healthy eating. Follow these and you will be eating a healthy diet without even thinking about it.

If you're trying to lose weight or just want to eat a controlled number of calories for weight maintenance, you'll find these 1,200-calorie and 1,600-calorie eating plans easy to follow. The menus are compiled from recipes in this book, along with many generic foods likely to be in your pantry or refrigerator. (Page numbers for recipes are included for your convenience.)

Substituting a food that is not on the menu (for example, baked potatoes instead of cooked rice) is no problem. Just check the Calorie/Nutrient Chart on pages 136 through 140 to find out how many calories the substitution contains.

Most women can safely lose weight by eating 1,200 calories a day, and most men can do the same at 1,600 calories a day. Feel free to use these menus for the entire family—not just the dieters. You can easily alter the meal by adding other healthy foods as side dishes or snacks, or plan for the nondieters to eat larger portions of food, if desired.

If those extra pounds come off slowly and you find yourself impatient, resist the urge to cut more calories to try to lose weight faster. Increase your exercise time instead. (See page 14 for calorie-burning exercise suggestions.) Severely restricting calories may rob your body of the nutrients you need to stay healthy. And it can cause your metabolism to slow down to accommodate a limited food supply. When that happens, you may be more likely to regain the weight you've lost (and more) when you go back to a normal diet.

DAY 1

BREAKFAST
Raisin Bread French Toast with Apple Syrup (page 24)	134
½ cup cooked grits or oatmeal	73
½ cup unsweetened grapefruit juice	47
	254

LUNCH
Garden Turkey Pocket (page 53)	184
1 medium pear	97
1 cup skim milk	86
	367

SUPPER
Pasta with Canadian Bacon (page 75)	257
2 cups romaine lettuce with 2 tablespoons nonfat Italian dressing	34
½ (2-ounce) plain or onion bagel	81
1 cup skim milk	86
	458

SNACK
3 (2½-inch) squares graham crackers	90
1 teaspoon reduced-fat peanut butter	30
TOTAL CALORIES	**1,199**

(CALORIES FROM FAT: 10%)

1,600-CALORIE DIET
Add: 2 slices turkey bacon, 1 cup Tropical Fruit Smoothie (page 119), ½ bagel, ½ cup chocolate nonfat ice cream, and 1 square graham cracker.
(CALORIES FROM FAT: 11%)

Super-Quick Menu Ideas

What about those days when you're really busy and only have time for a quick bagel or sandwich? Don't use that as an excuse to abandon your meal plan.

Just substitute one of the breakfast, lunch, or snack ideas on the following pages for the scheduled meal. Calories are provided for each to help you stay on track.

Day 2

Breakfast
3 Sausage and Cheese Biscuits (page 18)	198
1 cup cubed cantaloupe	56
½ cup skim milk	43
	297

Lunch
Mushroom and Roasted Pepper Sandwich (page 63)	225
1 ounce plain bagel chips	70
1 medium orange	62
	357

Supper
Oriental Tuna Patty (page 87)	131
Seasoned Vermicelli and Rice (page 83)	141
½ cup steamed snow peas	34
½ (6-inch) whole wheat pita bread, toasted	61
1 cup fresh or frozen blueberries	82
	449

Snack
½ cup coffee-flavored low-fat yogurt	97
TOTAL CALORIES	**1,200**

(Calories from Fat: 15%)

1,600-Calorie Diet
Add: ½ cup skim milk, ½ cup snow peas, ½ pita bread, 1 teaspoon reduced-calorie margarine, 1 (2-ounce) slice angel food cake, and ½ cup coffee-flavored low-fat yogurt.
(Calories from Fat: 14%)

Day 3

Breakfast
1 (2-ounce) plain bagel	161
2 tablespoons nonfat cream cheese	24
½ cup unsweetened orange juice	56
	241

Lunch
Easy Sloppy Joe (page 45)	272
1 kiwifruit	44
1 cup skim milk	86
	402

Supper
Simple Baked Chicken (page 80)	235
½ cup cooked barley	97
½ cup cooked baby carrots	33
1 (1-ounce) whole wheat roll	72
½ cup unsweetened fruit cocktail or assorted fresh fruit	57
	494

Snack
¾ cup tomato juice	31
3 unsalted crackers	30
TOTAL CALORIES	**1,198**

(Calories from Fat: 14%)

1,600-Calorie Diet
Add: 2 Almond Biscotti (page 130), ½ cup barley, 1 (1-ounce) whole wheat roll, 1½ teaspoons reduced-calorie margarine, and ½ cup fruit cocktail.
(Calories from Fat: 17%)

Quick Breakfasts

- 260 calories (11% fat): 1 cup cooked farina, 1 ounce Canadian bacon, ½ cup fresh strawberries, 1 cup skim milk

- 270 calories (25% fat): 1 poached egg, 1 slice whole wheat toast, 1 teaspoon reduced-calorie margarine, ½ cup grits, ½ cup unsweetened grapefruit juice

- 273 calories (7% fat): ½ cup whole bran cereal, 1 cup skim milk, 1 tablespoon raisins, ½ cup unsweetened orange juice

- 280 calories (18% fat): ¼ cup egg substitute (cooked), 2 slices turkey bacon, 2 slices toasted raisin bread, ½ cup unsweetened apple juice

- 292 calories (13% fat): 1 toasted English muffin, 1 tablespoon reduced-calorie fruit jam, ½ cup fresh pineapple chunks, ½ cup skim milk

- 294 calories (6% fat): 1 (2-ounce) plain bagel, 2 tablespoons nonfat cream cheese, 1 banana

- 322 calories (16% fat): 1 cup vanilla low-fat yogurt, 1 slice whole wheat toast, 1 teaspoon reduced-calorie margarine, 1 cup cubed cantaloupe

DAY 4

BREAKFAST
1 Raspberry-Filled Cinnamon Muffin (page 19)	153
½ grapefruit	39
1 cup skim milk	86
	278

LUNCH
Southwestern Chicken Salad Sandwich (page 49)	225
20 thin pretzels	50
1 banana	109
	384

SUPPER
Pork Madeira (page 102)	155
Mashed Potatoes (page 102)	119
1 cup steamed broccoli	24
1 (1-ounce) slice French bread	73
½ cup strawberry nonfat frozen yogurt	82
	453

SNACK
Orange-Pineapple Slush (page 121)	86
TOTAL CALORIES	**1,201**

(CALORIES FROM FAT: 13%)

1,600-CALORIE DIET
Add: 1 Raspberry-Filled Cinnamon Muffin, 10 thin pretzels, 3 gingersnaps, 1½ teaspoons reduced-calorie margarine, and 1 cup skim milk.
(CALORIES FROM FAT: 18%)

DAY 5

BREAKFAST
1 slice Raisin-Bran Loaf (page 23)	136
½ cup vanilla low-fat yogurt	97
1 cup fresh strawberries	45
	278

LUNCH
Chef's Salad: 2 cups mixed salad greens	16
1 ounce reduced-fat ham	35
1 ounce reduced-fat Cheddar cheese	71
2 tablespoons nonfat Italian dressing	16
1 (6-inch) whole wheat pita bread, toasted	122
1 apple	81
	341

SUPPER
Grouper Fingers with Lemon-Pepper Mayonnaise (page 85)	147
1 cup cooked couscous	200
1 cup steamed spinach	42
1 (1-ounce) whole wheat roll	72
1½ teaspoons reduced-calorie margarine	26
	487

SNACK
Tropical Frozen Yogurt (page 86)	97
TOTAL CALORIES	**1,203**

(CALORIES FROM FAT: 14%)

1,600-CALORIE DIET
Add: 1 slice Raisin Bran Loaf, ½ cup vanilla low-fat yogurt, 1 (1-ounce) roll, and 1 cup skim milk.
(CALORIES FROM FAT: 15%)

QUICK LUNCHES

- 312 calories (23% fat): ½ cup nonfat cottage cheese, 1 medium peach, 1 cup Bibb lettuce, 6 whole wheat crackers (about 1½ ounces)

- 315 calories (6% fat): Sandwich [2 ounces canned tuna in water, 1 tablespoon chopped sweet pickle, 2 teaspoons nonfat mayonnaise, 1 (6-inch) whole wheat pita bread] and 1 medium pear

- 316 calories (24% fat): Chef's salad (2 cups romaine lettuce, 1 ounce reduced-fat Cheddar cheese, 1 ounce roasted turkey breast, 2 tablespoons nonfat Italian salad dressing), 5 commercial breadsticks, 1 cup fresh blueberries

- 325 calories (24% fat): Sandwich (2 slices whole wheat bread, 2 ounces reduced-fat ham, 1 lettuce leaf, 2 teaspoons reduced-calorie mayonnaise), 1 orange, 20 thin pretzel sticks

- 326 calories (14% fat): 1 cup vanilla low-fat yogurt, 1 cup fresh strawberries, 8 plain melba rounds

- 345 calories (22% fat): Sandwich (2 slices whole wheat bread, 1 tablespoon reduced-fat peanut butter), 1 cup skim milk, ½ cup seedless grapes

DAY 6

BREAKFAST
4 Silver Dollar Pancakes (page 31)	160
2 tablespoons reduced-calorie maple syrup	60
1 cup skim milk	86
	306

LUNCH
Grilled New Yorker (page 55)	276
1 cup celery sticks	20
1 cup fresh or canned unsweetened peaches	58
	354

SUPPER
Mama's Chicken Stew (page 79)	257
Poppy Seed Coleslaw (page 73)	36
1 (1-ounce) slice French bread	73
1 teaspoon reduced-calorie margarine	17
Fresh Fruit with Strawberry Sauce (page 132)	99
	482

SNACK
½ cup seedless grapes	57
TOTAL CALORIES	**1,199**

(CALORIES FROM FAT: 13%)

1,600-CALORIE DIET
Add: 2 Silver Dollar Pancakes, 1 (1-ounce) slice French bread, ½ cup vanilla nonfat ice cream, 1 cup skim milk, and ½ cup seedless grapes.
(CALORIES FROM FAT: 11%)

DAY 7

BREAKFAST
1 Apricot Scone (page 130)	149
½ grapefruit	39
1 cup skim milk	86
	274

LUNCH
White Bean-Vegetable Salad (page 59)	278
5 plain melba rounds	55
½ cup fresh pineapple chunks	38
	371

SUPPER
Grilled Sirloin with Sweet Red Pepper Sauce (page 96)	201
1 small baked potato	110
2 tablespoons nonfat sour cream	20
1 cup steamed zucchini	34
2 (1-ounce) slices Italian bread	146
	511

SNACK
2 cups hot-air popped popcorn	46
TOTAL CALORIES	**1,202**

(CALORIES FROM FAT: 17%)

1,600-CALORIE DIET
Add: 1 Apricot Scone, ½ cup pineapple chunks, 1 cup skim milk, and 1 cup Spiced Orange Cider (page 118).
(CALORIES FROM FAT: 16%)

QUICK SNACKS

- 0 to 10 calories: 1 cup coffee or tea OR ½ cup raw celery sticks OR ½ cup sliced raw zucchini
- 11 to 20 calories: ½ cup raw broccoli OR ½ cup raw cauliflower OR 1 medium-size sweet pepper
- 21 to 30 calories: 1 cup hot-air popped popcorn OR 10 thin pretzel sticks OR 1 medium tomato
- 31 to 40 calories: 1 medium-size raw carrot OR 1 medium cucumber OR 1 plain rice cake
- 41 to 50 calories: 1 cup tomato juice OR 1 kiwifruit OR 1 cup fresh strawberries OR 1 ounce low-fat process American cheese OR ½ cup fresh blueberries
- 51 to 60 calories: 1 cup melon OR ½ cup unsweetened fruit cocktail OR ½ cup seedless grapes
- 61 to 70 calories: 1 medium orange OR 2 whole wheat crackers OR 1 fresh nectarine OR 4 vanilla wafers OR 6 plain melba rounds
- 71 to 80 calories: 2 gingersnaps OR 1 cup fresh pineapple chunks OR 1 (1-ounce) slice angel food cake
- 81 to 90 calories: 1 medium apple OR ½ (2-ounce) plain bagel OR ½ cup nonfat frozen yogurt
- 91 to 100 calories: ½ English muffin OR 1 medium pear OR ½ cup vanilla nonfat ice cream

Think Trim and Healthy

Here are some basic strategies to help you keep a positive attitude while trying to lose weight:

• Make a list of all the healthy reasons for losing weight so that your goal is to feel good as well as to look good.

• Limit high-calorie foods you love but don't eliminate them. Just eat them less often and in smaller portions. Don't deprive yourself and then binge.

• Dish up a single serving at meals and immediately refrigerate leftovers—no second helpings.

• Avoid the starve-all-day, stuff-yourself-at-night routine. Eat at least three main meals to keep your appetite under control.

• Keep a food diary to find out what triggers you to overeat. Once you figure out the cause, it's easier to change unhealthy habits.

• Start thinking of eating as a balancing act. It's okay to indulge on occasion if you cut back at the following meal or the next day.

• Make small portions of food look larger by serving them on salad plates instead of dinner plates.

• Rethink the clean-your-plate directive. It's better to throw out the last few bites than to consume extra calories when you're not really hungry.

• Opt for a long-term commitment. Because it's either too much food or too little activity (or a combination of both) that causes weight gain, successful weight loss requires the development of new behaviors such as the strategies discussed. Too many dieters follow a weight loss plan or exercise program for only a short time, and then they resume their old habits. Changes need to be permanent if weight loss is to be permanent.

What about Exercise?

Don't forget that the cornerstone of a healthy lifestyle and weight-loss plan is exercise. As a major fat burner, exercise slows the loss of muscle tissue and boosts the metabolic rate (the rate at which you burn calories). If you diet without exercising, your body will burn muscle tissue. What's more, your body will lower its metabolic rate in an effort to protect itself from starvation.

Pick an activity you like and do it on a regular basis. Or better yet, pick a few activities that are fun for you. The variety will help keep you motivated and interested.

Walking is an excellent choice for beginners—it requires little skill, no elaborate equipment, and can be done almost anywhere. As you adapt to the exercise, you can make it more challenging by increasing your pace and level of intensity.

Using exercise equipment is another fitness alternative that doesn't call for a lot of skill yet offers a first-rate workout. Machines such as a treadmill, stationary bicycle, and stair stepper are convenient and easy to use; they also provide excellent cardiovascular benefits while toning muscles.

Calorie Burners

If you are trying to decide on an activity to keep you fit, it's helpful to know how much calorie-burning benefit each offers. Here's a guide to an hour's worth of a few activities:

Activity (one hour)	Body Weight/Calories Burned			
	120 lbs.	150 lbs.	180 lbs.	220 lbs.
Cycling 6 mph	192	240	282	360
Walking 3 mph	198	246	294	360
Swimming 1 mph	312	396	480	585
Cross-country skiing 4 mph	468	474	714	870
Running 5½ mph	480	600	702	888

LOW-FAT BASICS

Whether you are trying to lose or maintain weight, low-fat eating makes good sense. Research studies show that decreasing your fat intake reduces risks of heart disease, diabetes, and some types of cancer. The goal recommended by major health groups is an intake of 30 percent or less of total daily calories.

The *Low-Fat Ways To Cook* series helps you meet that goal. Each book gives you practical, delicious recipes with realistic advice about low-fat cooking and eating. The recipes are lower in total fat than traditional recipes, and most provide less than 30 percent of calories from fat and less than 10 percent from saturated fat.

If you have one high-fat item during a meal, you can balance it with low-fat choices for the rest of the day and still remain within the recommended percentage. For example, fat contributes 46 percent of the calories in Tossed Salad Supremo for the Make-Ahead Dinner beginning on page 108. However, because the salad is combined with other low-fat foods, the total menu provides only 23 percent of calories as fat.

The goal of fat reduction is not to eliminate fat entirely. In fact, some fat is needed to transport fat-soluble vitamins and maintain other body functions.

FIGURING THE FAT

The easiest way to achieve a diet with 30 percent or fewer of total calories from fat is to establish a daily "fat budget" based on the total number of calories you need each day. To estimate your daily calorie requirements, multiply your current weight by 15. Remember that this is only a rough guide because calorie requirements vary according to age, body size, and level of activity. To gain or lose 1 pound a week, add or subtract 500 calories a day. (A diet of fewer than 1,200 calories a day is not recommended unless medically supervised.)

Once you determine your calorie requirement, it's easy to figure the number of fat grams you should consume each day. These should equal or be lower than the number of fat grams indicated on the Daily Fat Limits chart.

DAILY FAT LIMITS		
Calories Per Day	30 Percent of Calories	Grams of Fat
1,200	360	40
1,500	450	50
1,800	540	60
2,000	600	67
2,200	660	73
2,500	750	83
2,800	840	93

NUTRITIONAL ANALYSIS

Each recipe in *Low-Fat Ways To Lose Weight* has been kitchen-tested by a staff of qualified home economists. Registered dietitians have determined the nutrient information, using a computer system that analyzes every ingredient. These efforts ensure the success of each recipe and will help you fit these recipes into your own meal planning.

The nutrient grid that follows each recipe provides calories per serving and the percentage of calories from fat. Also, the grid lists the grams of total fat, saturated fat, protein, and carbohydrate, and the milligrams of cholesterol and sodium per serving. The nutrient values are as accurate as possible and are based on these assumptions.

• When the recipe calls for cooked pasta, rice, or noodles, we base the analysis on cooking without additional salt or fat.

• The calculations indicate that meat and poultry are trimmed of fat and skin before cooking.

• Only the amount of marinade absorbed by the food is calculated.

• Garnishes and other optional ingredients are not calculated.

• Some of the alcohol calories evaporate during heating, and only those remaining are calculated.

• When a range is given for an ingredient (3 to 3½ cups, for instance), we calculate the lesser amount.

• Fruits and vegetables listed in the ingredients are not peeled unless specified.

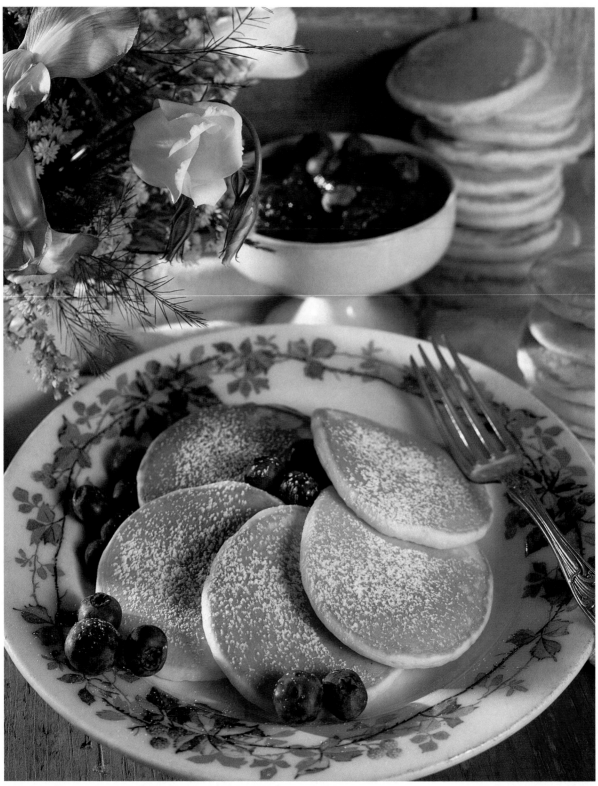

Silver Dollar Pancakes and Blueberry Applesauce (menu on page 31)

BREAKFASTS & BRUNCHES

*L*ow-fat cooking has transformed the look of today's breakfast. Now you can enjoy biscuits (pages 18 and 21), pancakes (page 31), and even French toast (page 24) yet still keep your calories and fat to a healthy minimum.

If you like to start your morning with eggs, you're in luck. Hearty Omelet (page 27) and Scrambled Breakfast Sandwiches (page 30) take advantage of egg substitutes to keep cholesterol low.

For mornings when you have more time to cook, try the menu featuring Crabmeat Crêpes (beginning on page 35). It serves eight and is perfect for a company brunch.

BISCUITS TO GO

Servings		*Calories*
3 biscuits	Sausage and Cheese Biscuits	198
½ cup	Orange juice	56

Serves 4
TOTAL CALORIES PER SERVING: 254
(CALORIES FROM FAT: 25%)

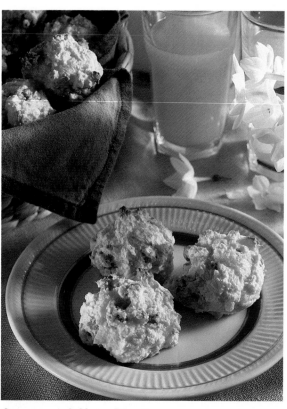

Sausage and Cheese Biscuits

SAUSAGE AND CHEESE BISCUITS

¼ pound raw turkey sausage
½ cup all-purpose flour
½ cup unprocessed oat bran
½ cup (2 ounces) shredded reduced-fat
    Cheddar cheese
1 teaspoon baking powder
⅛ teaspoon baking soda
½ cup plus 3 tablespoons nonfat buttermilk
Vegetable cooking spray

  Place sausage in a nonstick skillet; cook over medium heat until browned, stirring until it crumbles. Drain and pat dry with paper towels.
  Combine sausage, flour, and next 4 ingredients in a bowl; stir well. Add buttermilk, stirring just until moistened. Drop dough by heaping tablespoonfuls onto a baking sheet coated with cooking spray. Bake at 450° for 11 minutes. Yield: 1 dozen.

PER BISCUIT: 66 CALORIES (31% FROM FAT)
FAT 2.3G (SATURATED FAT 0.6G)
PROTEIN 4.6G   CARBOHYDRATE 6.8G
CHOLESTEROL 9MG   SODIUM 110MG

Fat Alert

  When you start the day with biscuits from a fast-food restaurant, you're probably getting a hefty load of calories and fat. Here's a better solution. Make Sausage and Cheese Biscuits the night before. Then in the morning, heat the biscuits while you dress. Enjoy with a glass of orange juice or take the biscuits with you for a meal that's lower in fat than the drive-through variety.

MORNING MUFFINS

Servings		*Calories*
1 muffin	Raspberry-Filled Cinnamon Muffins	153
1 serving	Minted Fruit Compote	70
1 cup	Skim milk	86

Serves 6
TOTAL CALORIES PER SERVING: 309
(CALORIES FROM FAT: 15%)

RASPBERRY-FILLED CINNAMON MUFFINS

1½ cups all-purpose flour
2½ teaspoons baking powder
¼ teaspoon salt
1 teaspoon ground cinnamon
½ cup sugar
⅔ cup low-fat buttermilk
¼ cup margarine, melted
1 egg, lightly beaten
Vegetable cooking spray
¼ cup seedless raspberry preserves
1 tablespoon sugar
¼ teaspoon ground cinnamon

Combine first 5 ingredients in a medium bowl, and make a well in center of mixture. Combine buttermilk, margarine, and egg, and stir well. Add to flour mixture, stirring just until moistened.

Spoon about 1 tablespoon batter into each of 12 muffin cups coated with cooking spray. Spoon 1 teaspoon preserves into center of each muffin cup, and top with remaining batter.

Combine 1 tablespoon sugar and ¼ teaspoon cinnamon; stir well. Sprinkle evenly over muffins. Bake at 400° for 20 minutes or until muffins spring back when touched lightly in center. Remove muffins from pans immediately, and place on a wire rack. Yield: 1 dozen.

PER MUFFIN: 153 CALORIES (27% FROM FAT)
FAT 4.6G (SATURATED FAT 1.0G)
PROTEIN 2.6G CARBOHYDRATE 25.7G
CHOLESTEROL 18MG SODIUM 116MG

MINTED FRUIT COMPOTE

4 medium oranges, peeled, sectioned, and seeded
1½ cups pink grapefruit sections
1 cup sliced fresh strawberries
1 tablespoon chopped fresh mint
2 teaspoons sugar
Fresh mint sprigs (optional)

Combine first 5 ingredients in a large bowl; stir to mix. Cover and chill thoroughly.

To serve, spoon fruit mixture evenly into 6 dessert glasses. Garnish each with fresh mint sprigs, if desired. Serve chilled. Yield: 6 servings.

PER SERVING: 70 CALORIES (3% FROM FAT)
FAT 0.2G (SATURATED FAT 0.0G)
PROTEIN 1.3G CARBOHYDRATE 17.4G
CHOLESTEROL 0MG SODIUM 0MG

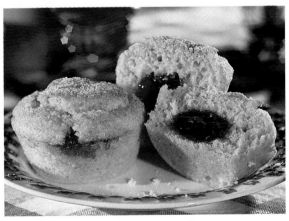

Raspberry-Filled Cinnamon Muffins

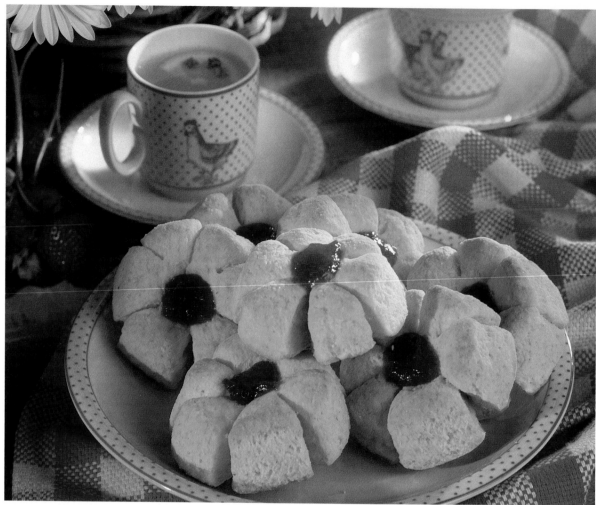

Cornmeal Daisy Biscuits

DOWN-HOME SOUTHERN BREAKFAST

Servings		*Calories*
2 biscuits	Cornmeal Daisy Biscuits	156
2 slices	Turkey bacon	61
1 serving	Sweet Potato Browns	104
¾ cup	Warm Apple Lemonade	86

Serves 6

TOTAL CALORIES PER SERVING: 407
(CALORIES FROM FAT: 22%)

CORNMEAL DAISY BISCUITS

1½ cups all-purpose flour
½ cup cornmeal
2 teaspoons baking powder
¼ teaspoon baking soda
¼ teaspoon salt
1 tablespoon sugar
3 tablespoons margarine
¾ cup nonfat buttermilk
1 tablespoon all-purpose flour
1½ tablespoons reduced-calorie strawberry
   preserves

Combine first 6 ingredients in a medium bowl; cut in margarine with a pastry blender until mixture resembles coarse meal. Add buttermilk, stirring just until dry ingredients are moistened.

Sprinkle 1 tablespoon flour over work surface. Turn dough out onto surface, and knead 3 or 4 times. Roll dough to ½-inch thickness; cut into rounds using a 2-inch biscuit cutter.

Place rounds on an ungreased baking sheet. Cut six ½-inch slashes evenly around edge of each biscuit to form petals. Press thumb in center of each biscuit, leaving an indentation. Place ¼ teaspoon preserves in each indentation. Bake at 425° for 10 minutes or until lightly browned. Yield: 1½ dozen.

PER BISCUIT: 78 CALORIES (24% FROM FAT)
FAT 2.1G (SATURATED FAT 0.4G)
PROTEIN 1.8G   CARBOHYDRATE 12.8G
CHOLESTEROL 0MG   SODIUM 111MG

Lighten Up

After years of rejection by dedicated dieters, bacon is back on the menu. But today's alternative to regular bacon is turkey bacon. It scales in at only 106 calories and 7 grams of fat per ounce compared to 163 calories and 14 grams of fat in regular bacon.

SWEET POTATO BROWNS

Butter-flavored vegetable cooking spray
1½ teaspoons margarine
3 cups peeled, shredded sweet potato (about
   2½ medium)
1½ cups peeled, diced Granny Smith apple
3 tablespoons minced onion
1 tablespoon brown sugar
¼ teaspoon ground allspice
3 tablespoons unsweetened apple juice

Coat a large nonstick skillet with cooking spray; add margarine. Place over medium-high heat until margarine melts. Add potato, apple, and onion; sauté 5 minutes.

Add brown sugar, allspice, and apple juice; cook, stirring constantly, 5 minutes or until potato is tender. Serve immediately. Yield: 6 servings.

PER SERVING: 104 CALORIES (12% FROM FAT)
FAT 1.4G (SATURATED FAT 0.3G)
PROTEIN 1.1G   CARBOHYDRATE 22.6G
CHOLESTEROL 0MG   SODIUM 20MG

WARM APPLE LEMONADE

2¾ cups water
1¼ cups unsweetened apple juice
¾ cup fresh lemon juice
¼ cup plus 1 tablespoon honey
¼ teaspoon ground nutmeg
3 whole allspice
3 whole cloves
1 (3-inch) stick cinnamon
Lemon slices studded with whole cloves
   (optional)

Combine first 8 ingredients in a medium saucepan; bring to a boil. Reduce heat, and simmer, uncovered, 10 minutes. Remove and discard whole spices. Pour into individual mugs; top with lemon slices, if desired. Yield: 6 (¾-cup) servings.

PER SERVING: 86 CALORIES (1% FROM FAT)
FAT 0.1G (SATURATED FAT 0.0G)
PROTEIN 0.2G   CARBOHYDRATE 23.3G
CHOLESTEROL 0MG   SODIUM 3MG

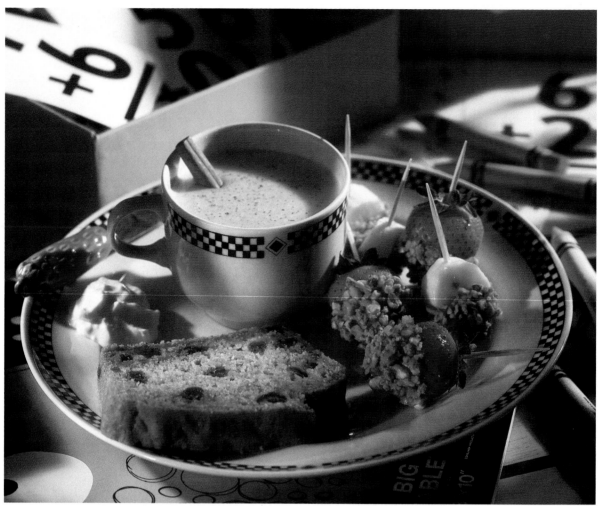

Vanilla-Almond Milk, Frosty Fruit, Raisin-Bran Loaf, and Apple-Maple Spread

FIRST DAY OF SCHOOL

Servings		*Calories*
1 slice	Raisin-Bran Loaf	136
1 tablespoon	Apple-Maple Spread	30
1 serving	Frosty Fruit	125
¾ cup	Vanilla-Almond Milk	121

Serves 4
TOTAL CALORIES PER SERVING: 412
(CALORIES FROM FAT: 19%)

RAISIN-BRAN LOAF

2½ cups wheat bran flakes cereal, divided
½ cup hot water
3 tablespoons vegetable oil
1½ cups all-purpose flour
1 teaspoon baking powder
1 teaspoon baking soda
½ teaspoon ground cinnamon
¼ teaspoon ground nutmeg
⅓ cup firmly packed brown sugar
1 cup nonfat buttermilk
¼ cup frozen egg substitute, thawed
2 teaspoons grated orange rind
½ cup raisins
Vegetable cooking spray

Combine 1½ cups cereal, water, and oil; set aside.
Combine flour and next 5 ingredients in a large bowl; make a well in center of mixture. Combine buttermilk, egg substitute, and orange rind; add to dry ingredients, stirring just until moistened. Stir in cereal mixture, remaining 1 cup cereal, and raisins.
Spoon batter into an 8½- x 4½- x 3-inch loafpan coated with cooking spray. Bake at 350° for 55 minutes or until a wooden pick inserted in center comes out clean. Let cool in pan on a wire rack 10 minutes; remove from pan, and let cool completely. Yield: 16 (½-inch) slices.

PER SLICE: 136 CALORIES (20% FROM FAT)
FAT 3.0G (SATURATED FAT 0.6G)
PROTEIN 3.5G   CARBOHYDRATE 25.5G
CHOLESTEROL 1MG   SODIUM 177MG

APPLE-MAPLE SPREAD

1 cup apple-cinnamon low-fat yogurt
½ cup light process cream cheese, softened
2 tablespoons reduced-calorie maple syrup

Spoon yogurt onto several layers of heavy-duty paper towels, spreading to ½-inch thickness. Cover with additional paper towels; let stand 5 minutes.
Beat cream cheese in a small bowl at medium speed of an electric mixer until creamy. Add yogurt to cream cheese, scraping yogurt from towels using a rubber spatula. Add syrup, stirring well. Cover and chill until ready to serve. Yield: 1 cup.

PER TABLESPOON: 30 CALORIES (39% FROM FAT)
FAT 1.3G (SATURATED FAT 0.8G)
PROTEIN 1.3G   CARBOHYDRATE 3.3G
CHOLESTEROL 5MG   SODIUM 48MG

FROSTY FRUIT

¼ cup nutlike cereal nuggets
3 tablespoons finely chopped pecans, toasted
12 fresh strawberries
1 medium banana, peeled and cut into 12 slices
24 wooden picks
⅓ cup strawberry-banana low-fat yogurt

Combine cereal and pecans; set aside. Place fruit on wooden picks; dip in yogurt, coating halfway up sides of fruit. Roll yogurt-coated portion of fruit in cereal mixture. Place on a baking sheet lined with wax paper. Cover; freeze 45 minutes. Yield: 4 servings.

PER SERVING: 125 CALORIES (30% FROM FAT)
FAT 4.2G (SATURATED FAT 0.5G)
PROTEIN 2.6G   CARBOHYDRATE 21.5G
CHOLESTEROL 1MG   SODIUM 60MG

VANILLA-ALMOND MILK

3 cups skim milk
3 tablespoons honey
2 teaspoons vanilla extract
¼ teaspoon almond extract
Ground nutmeg (optional)
Cinnamon sticks (optional)

Combine first 4 ingredients in a small saucepan. Cook over medium-low heat just until thoroughly heated, stirring frequently. Pour into serving mugs. If desired, sprinkle with nutmeg, and garnish with cinnamon sticks. Yield: 4 (¾-cup) servings.

PER SERVING: 121 CALORIES (2% FROM FAT)
FAT 0.3G (SATURATED FAT 0.2G)
PROTEIN 6.3G   CARBOHYDRATE 22.7G
CHOLESTEROL 4MG   SODIUM 96MG

BREAKFAST IN THE GREAT OUTDOORS

Servings		_Calories_
1 serving	Raisin French Toast with Apple Syrup	134
2 links	Spicy Pork Sausage	72
1 serving	Grilled Oranges and Grapefruit	67
1 cup	Hot coffee	5

Serves 4

TOTAL CALORIES PER SERVING: 278
(CALORIES FROM FAT: 20%)

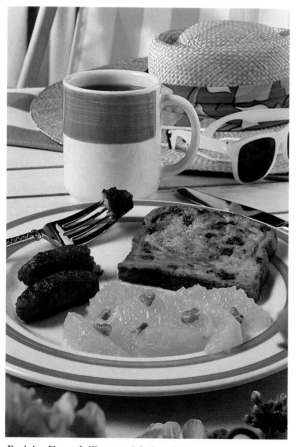

Raisin French Toast with Apple Syrup, Grilled Oranges and Grapefruit, and Spicy Pork Sausage

RAISIN FRENCH TOAST WITH APPLE SYRUP

¼ cup unsweetened apple cider
2 tablespoons low-sugar apple jelly
1 tablespoon brown sugar
½ teaspoon cornstarch
Vegetable cooking spray
½ cup plus 2 tablespoons frozen egg substitute, thawed
¼ cup skim milk
½ teaspoon vanilla extract
4 (1-ounce) slices cinnamon-raisin bread

Combine first 4 ingredients in a saucepan. Place grill rack over medium-hot coals (350° to 400°). Place saucepan on rack; cook, stirring constantly, until jelly melts and mixture is slightly thickened. Remove from heat; set aside, and keep warm.

Coat a 10-inch cast-iron skillet with cooking spray; place on rack until hot. Combine egg substitute, milk, and vanilla in a bowl. Dip 2 bread slices in egg mixture. Place in skillet; cook, covered, 5 to 7 minutes on each side or until browned. Repeat with remaining bread and egg mixture. Serve warm with cider mixture. Yield: 4 servings.

Note: French toast and syrup can be prepared conventionally. Cook syrup in a saucepan over medium heat until jelly melts and mixture is slightly thickened; set aside, and keep warm. Cook dipped bread slices in a large skillet coated with cooking spray over medium heat 4 to 5 minutes on each side or until browned.

PER SERVING: 134 CALORIES (7% FROM FAT)
FAT 1.0G (SATURATED FAT 0.2G)
PROTEIN 6.2G CARBOHYDRATE 24.7G
CHOLESTEROL 1MG SODIUM 177MG

SPICY PORK SAUSAGE

If prepackaged lean ground pork is not available at your supermarket, ask the butcher to grind some lean pork loin for you.

⅓ pound lean ground pork
1½ tablespoons fine, dry breadcrumbs
1 tablespoon finely chopped onion
½ teaspoon ground sage
¼ teaspoon fennel seeds, crushed
¼ teaspoon ground thyme
¼ teaspoon hot sauce
⅛ teaspoon salt
⅛ teaspoon garlic powder
⅛ teaspoon ground red pepper
⅛ teaspoon black pepper
1 egg white, lightly beaten
Vegetable cooking spray

Combine first 12 ingredients in a medium bowl, stirring well. Shape mixture into 8 links.

Place grill rack on grill over medium-hot coals (350° to 400°). Coat a large cast-iron skillet with cooking spray, and place on rack until hot. Place sausage links in skillet, and cook 9 to 10 minutes or until browned, turning frequently. Drain links on paper towels. Serve warm. Yield: 8 links.

Note: Sausage can be cooked conventionally. Place links in a large skillet coated with cooking spray. Place over medium heat, and cook 8 to 10 minutes or until browned, turning frequently.

PER LINK: 36 CALORIES (38% FROM FAT)
FAT 1.5G (SATURATED FAT 0.5G)
PROTEIN 4.5G CARBOHYDRATE 1.0G
CHOLESTEROL 11MG SODIUM 63MG

GRILLED ORANGES AND GRAPEFRUIT

1 cup fresh grapefruit sections
1 cup fresh orange sections
1 tablespoon water
2½ teaspoons brown sugar
2 teaspoons reduced-calorie margarine, melted
2 teaspoons chopped pecans, toasted

Arrange grapefruit and orange sections evenly on one half of a large piece of heavy-duty aluminum foil. Combine water, brown sugar, and margarine; brush fruit evenly with brown sugar mixture. Sprinkle with pecans. Fold foil over fruit; crimp edges to seal.

Place grill rack on grill over medium-hot coals (350° to 400°). Place foil packet on rack; grill, covered, 1 to 2 minutes or until thoroughly heated.

To serve, remove fruit mixture from foil packet, and transfer to individual serving plates. Serve warm. Yield: 4 (½-cup) servings.

Note: Foil packet can be cooked conventionally. Place packet on a baking sheet, and bake at 425° for 10 minutes or until thoroughly heated.

PER SERVING: 67 CALORIES (30% FROM FAT)
FAT 2.2G (SATURATED FAT 0.2G)
PROTEIN 0.9G CARBOHYDRATE 12.5G
CHOLESTEROL 0MG SODIUM 19MG

Exercise Tip

Sure, you know exercise is good for your health. But sometimes that fact alone isn't enough to get you moving. Studies show that one of the best motivations for sticking to an exercise program is to exercise with someone else. So ask a friend or family member to be your partner. You'll both feel better and look better, and you'll reduce your health risks, too.

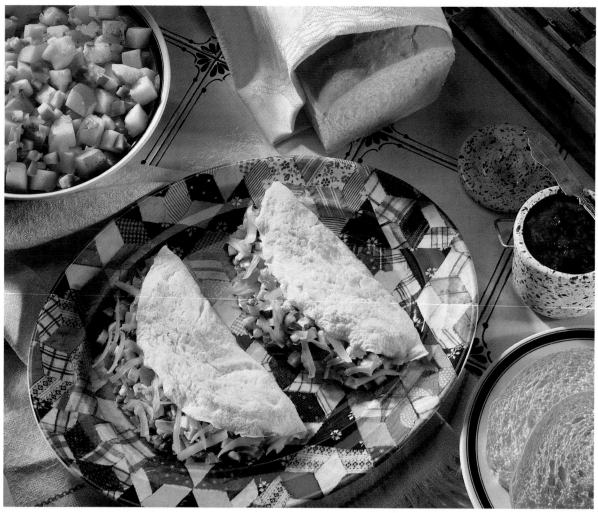

Hearty Omelet and Potato Medley

COUNTRY BREAKFAST

Servings		*Calories*
1 serving	Hearty Omelet	179
1 serving	Potato Medley	98
1 slice	Whole wheat toast	58
2 teaspoons	Reduced-calorie blackberry jam	19
1 serving	Broiled Grapefruit	104

Serves 4
TOTAL CALORIES PER SERVING: 458
(CALORIES FROM FAT: 20%)

HEARTY OMELET

If you don't have sweet red pepper on hand, just increase the green pepper to ¹/₂ cup.

Vegetable cooking spray
¾ cup diced tomato
⅔ cup diced cooked turkey breast
½ cup chopped zucchini
¼ cup chopped green pepper
¼ cup chopped sweet red pepper
¼ cup sliced green onions
1 tablespoon chopped fresh parsley
¼ teaspoon hot sauce
1½ cups frozen egg substitute with cheese, thawed
¼ cup skim milk
½ teaspoon minced fresh oregano
¼ teaspoon pepper
¼ cup (1 ounce) shredded reduced-fat Cheddar cheese, divided

Coat a nonstick skillet with cooking spray; place over medium-high heat until hot. Add diced tomato and next 7 ingredients; sauté until tender, and set aside.

Combine egg substitute, milk, oregano, and pepper in a small bowl.

Coat a small nonstick skillet with cooking spray; place over medium heat until hot enough to sizzle a drop of water. Pour half of egg substitute mixture into skillet. As mixture begins to cook, gently lift edges of omelet with a spatula, and tilt pan to allow uncooked portions to flow underneath.

When mixture is set, spoon half of vegetable mixture over half of omelet; sprinkle with 2 tablespoons cheese. Loosen omelet with spatula, and carefully fold in half. Carefully slide omelet onto a warm serving platter. Cut omelet into 2 pieces.

Repeat procedure with remaining egg mixture and cheese. Yield: 4 servings.

PER SERVING: 179 CALORIES (33% FROM FAT)
FAT 6.5G (SATURATED FAT 1.7G)
PROTEIN 21.6G CARBOHYDRATE 7.1G
CHOLESTEROL 30MG SODIUM 410MG

POTATO MEDLEY

1¾ cups cubed new potato
1½ cups water
1 cup diced cooking apple
1 tablespoon lemon juice
Vegetable cooking spray
2 teaspoons vegetable oil
½ cup chopped onion

Combine potato and water in a medium saucepan. Bring to a boil; cover, reduce heat, and simmer 10 minutes or until potato is almost tender. Drain well, and set aside.

Combine apple and lemon juice. Toss; set aside.

Coat a large nonstick skillet with cooking spray; add oil. Place over medium-high heat until hot. Add potato and onion; sauté until potato is lightly browned and onion is tender. Add reserved apple; cover and cook 1 minute. Uncover and cook an additional 2 minutes. Yield: 4 (½-cup) servings.

PER SERVING: 98 CALORIES (24% FROM FAT)
FAT 2.6G (SATURATED FAT 0.5G)
PROTEIN 1.6G CARBOHYDRATE 18.0G
CHOLESTEROL 0MG SODIUM 5MG

BROILED GRAPEFRUIT

2 large pink grapefruit
1 teaspoon sugar
¼ cup no-sugar-added strawberry spread
¼ cup vanilla low-fat yogurt

Cut grapefruit in half crosswise; remove seeds, and loosen sections. Place grapefruit, cut side up, on rack of a broiler pan.

Sprinkle each grapefruit half with ¼ teaspoon sugar. Spread 1 tablespoon strawberry spread over each half. Broil 5½ inches from heat (with electric oven door partially opened) 6 minutes or until thoroughly heated and sugar melts. Top each half with 1 tablespoon yogurt. Yield: 4 servings.

PER SERVING: 104 CALORIES (3% FROM FAT)
FAT 0.3G (SATURATED FAT 0.1G)
PROTEIN 1.6G CARBOHYDRATE 26.4G
CHOLESTEROL 1MG SODIUM 9MG

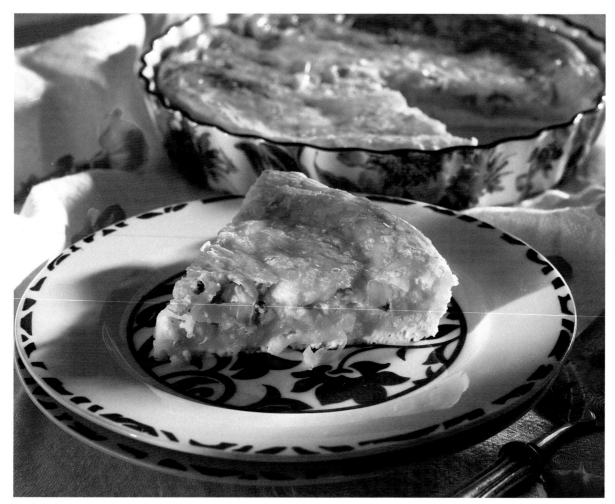

Quiche Lorraine

A LIGHTENED CLASSIC

Servings		*Calories*
1 serving	Quiche Lorraine	236
1 serving	Citrus Fruit Cocktail	84
½ bagel	Bagel	78
1 cup	Spiced Coffee	9

Serves 6

TOTAL CALORIES PER SERVING: 407
(CALORIES FROM FAT: 20%)

QUICHE LORRAINE

Using refrigerated breadstick dough for the pastry
makes this quiche especially easy.

1 (7-ounce) package refrigerated breadstick
    dough
Vegetable cooking spray
1½ cups slivered onion
6 slices turkey bacon, chopped
¾ cup (3 ounces) shredded reduced-fat
    reduced-sodium Swiss cheese
1 cup evaporated skimmed milk
2 teaspoons cornstarch
⅛ teaspoon ground nutmeg
Dash of ground red pepper
2 eggs
2 egg whites

Unroll breadstick dough, separating into strips.
Working on a flat surface, coil one strip of dough
around itself in a spiral pattern. Add second strip of
dough to the end of the first strip, pinching ends
together to seal; continue coiling dough in a spiral
pattern. Repeat procedure with remaining dough
strips to make an 8-inch flat circle. Roll dough into
a 13-inch circle, and fit into a 9-inch quiche dish or
pieplate coated with vegetable cooking spray. Fold
edges under, and flute; set prepared crust aside.

Combine onion and bacon in a medium nonstick
skillet coated with cooking spray. Cook over
medium-high heat 10 minutes, stirring frequently.
Spread onion mixture in prepared crust. Top onion
mixture with cheese, and set aside.

Combine milk and next 5 ingredients in container of an electric blender; cover and process
until smooth.

Pour milk mixture over cheese. Bake at 375° for
35 minutes or until a knife inserted 1 inch from
center comes out clean; let stand 10 minutes. To
serve, slice quiche into 6 wedges. Yield: 6 servings.

PER SERVING: 236 CALORIES (32% FROM FAT)
FAT 8.2G (SATURATED FAT 3.2G)
PROTEIN 16.1G CARBOHYDRATE 17.3G
CHOLESTEROL 94MG SODIUM 503MG

CITRUS FRUIT COCKTAIL

3 medium-size oranges, peeled, sectioned, and
    coarsely chopped
1 medium-size pink grapefruit, peeled,
    sectioned, and coarsely chopped
2 kiwifruit, peeled and coarsely chopped
¼ teaspoon grated orange rind
¼ teaspoon grated lime rind
3 tablespoons fresh orange juice
2 tablespoons honey
1 tablespoon fresh lime juice

Combine first 3 ingredients in a bowl; toss.
Combine orange rind and next 4 ingredients in a
bowl; stir until blended. Pour orange juice mixture
over fruit mixture; toss gently. Yield: 6 servings.

PER SERVING: 84 CALORIES (3% FROM FAT)
FAT 0.3G (SATURATED FAT 0.0G)
PROTEIN 1.3G CARBOHYDRATE 20.8G
CHOLESTEROL 0MG SODIUM 0MG

SPICED COFFEE

¾ cup ground Colombian coffee
¾ teaspoon ground cinnamon
¼ teaspoon ground nutmeg
2 teaspoons vanilla extract
8½ cups water

Place coffee in filter basket; sprinkle with cinnamon, nutmeg, and vanilla. Add water according to
manufacturer's instructions. Yield: 8 (1-cup) servings.

PER SERVING: 9 CALORIES (0% FROM FAT)
FAT 0.0G (SATURATED FAT 0.0G)
PROTEIN 0.2G CARBOHYDRATE 1.5G
CHOLESTEROL 0MG SODIUM 5MG

LAZY DAY BREAKFAST

Servings		*Calories*
1 serving	Scrambled Breakfast Sandwiches	163
1 serving	Sautéed Apple Rings with Orange Juice	70

Serves 4

TOTAL CALORIES PER SERVING: 233
(CALORIES FROM FAT: 18%)

SCRAMBLED BREAKFAST SANDWICHES

Vegetable cooking spray
¼ cup chopped sweet red pepper
1 tablespoon sliced green onions
½ cup frozen egg substitute, thawed
1 tablespoon grated Parmesan cheese
1 tablespoon skim milk
⅛ teaspoon dried Italian seasoning
Dash of ground white pepper
4 (¾-ounce) slices Canadian bacon
2 whole wheat English muffins, split and
   toasted
1 ounce reduced-fat Brie cheese, cubed

Coat a small nonstick skillet with cooking spray; place over medium-high heat until hot. Add sweet red pepper and green onions; sauté until tender.

Combine egg substitute and next 4 ingredients; beat well with a wire whisk. Pour over pepper mixture in skillet; cook over medium heat until egg substitute mixture is firm but still moist, stirring occasionally.

Place 1 slice of Canadian bacon on each muffin half. Spoon egg substitute mixture evenly over bacon, and top with cheese. Broil 5½ inches from heat (with electric oven door partially opened) 1 minute or until cheese melts. Serve immediately. Yield: 4 servings.

PER SERVING: 163 CALORIES (20% FROM FAT)
FAT 3.7G (SATURATED FAT 1.7G)
PROTEIN 12.3G CARBOHYDRATE 19.3G
CHOLESTEROL 18MG SODIUM 575MG

SAUTÉED APPLE RINGS WITH ORANGE JUICE

2 small Winesap apples
¼ cup unsweetened orange juice
1 tablespoon brown sugar
1 teaspoon ground cinnamon
1 teaspoon reduced-calorie margarine

Core apples, and slice each apple crosswise into 6 rings.

Combine orange juice and next 3 ingredients in a large nonstick skillet. Bring to a boil over medium heat, stirring until sugar dissolves. Arrange apple rings in skillet in a single layer. Cook 5 to 6 minutes or until tender, turning once. Serve warm. Yield: 4 servings.

PER SERVING: 70 CALORIES (12% FROM FAT)
FAT 0.9G (SATURATED FAT 0.1G)
PROTEIN 0.3G CARBOHYDRATE 16.9G
CHOLESTEROL 0MG SODIUM 10MG

Calorie Countdown

The next time you grab a bagel, consider its size. Although calorie-counting books often list the standard bagel at 2 ounces and 150 calories, many specialty bagels tip the scales at 4 to 5 ounces or more, boosting their counts to between 300 and 550 calories.

PASS THE PANCAKES

(pictured on page 16)

Servings		*Calories*
6 pancakes	Silver Dollar Pancakes	240
¼ cup	Blueberry Applesauce	48
1 slice	Sugared Turkey Bacon	78

Serves 6

TOTAL CALORIES PER SERVING: 366
(CALORIES FROM FAT: 16%)

SILVER DOLLAR PANCAKES

2 cups all-purpose flour
1 tablespoon baking powder
⅛ teaspoon salt
2 tablespoons sugar
1¼ cups skim milk
½ cup low-fat sour cream
2 egg whites, lightly beaten
1 egg, lightly beaten
Vegetable cooking spray
1 tablespoon sifted powdered sugar
Fresh blueberries (optional)

Combine first 4 ingredients in a medium bowl; make a well in center of mixture. Combine milk, sour cream, egg whites, and egg. Add milk mixture to dry ingredients, stirring just until dry ingredients are moistened.

Coat a nonstick griddle with cooking spray, and preheat to 350°. For each pancake, pour 1 heaping tablespoon batter onto hot griddle. Cook pancakes until tops are covered with bubbles and edges look cooked; turn pancakes, and cook other side.

Sprinkle pancakes with powdered sugar. Serve with Blueberry Applesauce, and garnish with fresh blueberries, if desired. Yield: 36 (2½-inch) pancakes.

PER PANCAKE: 40 CALORIES (14% FROM FAT)
FAT 0.6G (SATURATED FAT 0.3G)
PROTEIN 1.5G CARBOHYDRATE 6.9G
CHOLESTEROL 8MG SODIUM 19MG

BLUEBERRY APPLESAUCE

2 cups peeled, diced cooking apple
1 cup fresh or frozen blueberries, thawed
⅓ cup unsweetened orange juice
2 tablespoons sugar
1 teaspoon grated orange rind

Combine all ingredients in a saucepan. Bring to a boil; cover, reduce heat, and simmer 15 minutes. Place in food processor bowl. Process until almost smooth. Cover and chill. Yield: 1¾ cups.

PER TABLESPOON: 12 CALORIES (8% FROM FAT)
FAT 0.1G (SATURATED FAT 0.0G)
PROTEIN 0.1G CARBOHYDRATE 3.0G
CHOLESTEROL 0MG SODIUM 0MG

SUGARED TURKEY BACON

1 tablespoon brown sugar
1 tablespoon frozen egg substitute, thawed
1½ teaspoons low-sodium Worcestershire sauce
1½ teaspoons spicy brown mustard
6 slices turkey bacon
½ cup fine, dry breadcrumbs

Combine first 4 ingredients. Dip bacon into mixture; dredge in breadcrumbs. Place on rack of a broiler pan. Bake at 350° for 20 minutes. Yield: 6 slices.

PER SLICE: 78 CALORIES (30% FROM FAT)
FAT 2.6G (SATURATED FAT 0.6G)
PROTEIN 3.6G CARBOHYDRATE 9.0G
CHOLESTEROL 10MG SODIUM 307MG

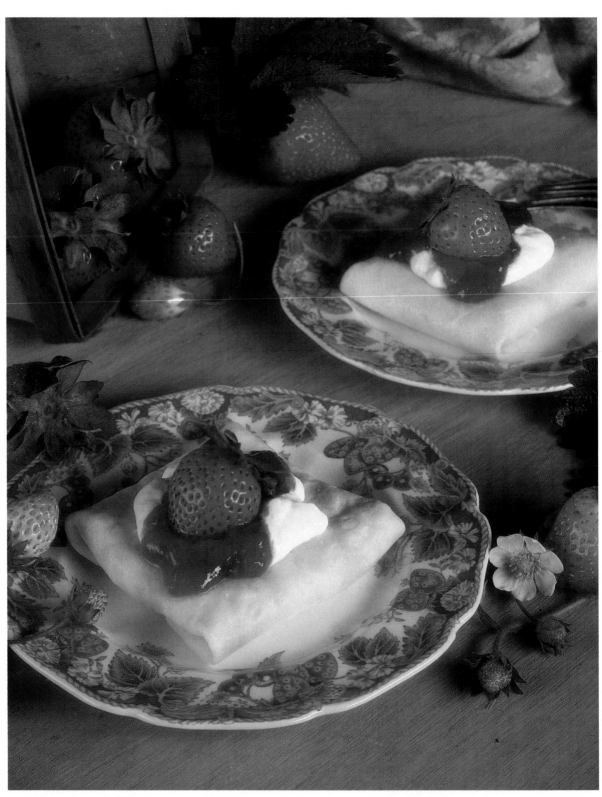

Strawberry-Cheese Blintzes

ELEGANT BEGINNING

Servings		Calories
2 blintzes	Strawberry-Cheese Blintzes	206
1 cup	Cubed honeydew	59
1 cup	Hot tea	2

Serves 6
TOTAL CALORIES PER SERVING: 267
(CALORIES FROM FAT: 18%)

STRAWBERRY-CHEESE BLINTZES

Blintzes filled with honey-sweetened cottage cheese and cream cheese make a special breakfast or brunch. Plan on two blintzes per serving.

1½ cups nonfat cottage cheese
½ cup light process cream cheese, softened
2 tablespoons honey
1 teaspoon grated lemon rind
½ teaspoon vanilla extract
2 egg whites, lightly beaten
12 Basic Crêpes
Vegetable cooking spray
¼ cup plus 2 tablespoons nonfat sour cream
¼ cup plus 2 tablespoons low-sugar
    strawberry spread
Fresh strawberries (optional)

Combine first 6 ingredients; stir well. Spoon 3 tablespoons cheese mixture in center of each Basic Crêpe. Fold right and left sides of crêpe over filling; fold bottom and top of crêpe over filling, forming a square.

Place blintzes, seam side down, on a large baking sheet coated with cooking spray. Bake at 350° for 12 minutes or until blintzes are thoroughly heated. To serve, place 2 blintzes on each of 6 individual plates. Top each serving with 1 tablespoon sour cream and 1 tablespoon strawberry spread. Garnish with fresh strawberries, if desired. Serve immediately. Yield: 12 blintzes.

BASIC CRÊPES

1⅓ cups all-purpose flour
¼ teaspoon salt
1½ cups plus 2 tablespoons skim milk
2 teaspoons vegetable oil
2 eggs, lightly beaten
2 egg whites, lightly beaten
Vegetable cooking spray

Combine flour and salt, stirring well. Combine milk, oil, eggs, and egg whites, stirring well. Gradually add milk mixture to flour mixture, beating well with a wire whisk until batter is smooth. Chill batter at least 2 hours.

Coat a 6-inch nonstick crêpe pan or skillet with cooking spray. Place over medium heat just until hot, not smoking. Pour 2 tablespoons batter into pan; quickly tilt pan in all directions so batter covers bottom of pan in a thin film. Cook 1 minute or until crêpe can be shaken loose from pan. Flip crêpe, and cook about 30 seconds. (Place filling on spotted side of crêpe.)

Place crêpes on a towel to cool. Stack cooled crêpes between layers of wax paper to prevent sticking. Repeat procedure until all batter is used. Yield: 2 dozen.

Note: Stack leftover crêpes between layers of wax paper, place in freezer bag, and freeze up to 1 month.

PER BLINTZ: 103 CALORIES (23% FROM FAT)
FAT 2.6G (SATURATED FAT 1.2G)
PROTEIN 8.2G   CARBOHYDRATE 12.4G
CHOLESTEROL 26MG   SODIUM 225MG

GOOD MORNING, SPRING

Servings		*Calories*
1 serving	Strawberry-Topped Puffy Pancake	217
1 serving	Poached Pineapple	129
1 cup	Iced coffee	5

Serves 4
TOTAL CALORIES PER SERVING: 351
(CALORIES FROM FAT: 11%)

STRAWBERRY-TOPPED PUFFY PANCAKE

½ cup 1% low-fat cottage cheese
¼ cup frozen orange juice concentrate, thawed and undiluted
2 tablespoons powdered sugar
⅔ cup skim milk
½ cup all-purpose flour
1 tablespoon honey
1 teaspoon grated lemon rind
2 eggs
Vegetable cooking spray
2⅓ cups halved fresh strawberries

Combine first 3 ingredients in container of an electric blender; cover and process until smooth. Spoon into a bowl; set aside.

Combine milk and next 4 ingredients in blender container; cover and process until smooth. Pour into a 9-inch pieplate coated with cooking spray. (Do not stir.)

Bake at 425° for 15 minutes or until puffed and golden. Spoon cottage cheese mixture onto pancake. Top with strawberries; cut into 4 wedges, and serve immediately. Yield: 4 servings.

PER SERVING: 217 CALORIES (15% FROM FAT)
FAT 3.6G (SATURATED FAT 1.1G)
PROTEIN 10.7G   CARBOHYDRATE 36.0G
CHOLESTEROL 112MG   SODIUM 171MG

POACHED PINEAPPLE

To make preparation a snap, buy peeled, cored fresh pineapple. You'll find it prepackaged in the produce section of the supermarket.

1 medium-size fresh pineapple, peeled and cored
1 cup unsweetened pineapple juice
2 tablespoons sugar
2 tablespoons lemon zest
¼ teaspoon whole cloves
1 (3-inch) stick cinnamon

Cut pineapple lengthwise into 12 spears, and set spears aside.

Combine pineapple juice and next 4 ingredients in a medium saucepan. Bring mixture to a boil over medium-high heat; cook, stirring constantly, until sugar dissolves. Reduce heat, and simmer, uncovered, 10 minutes.

Add pineapple spears. Bring to a boil; reduce heat, and simmer, uncovered, 8 minutes. Remove and discard cloves and cinnamon stick. Serve warm or chilled. Yield: 4 servings.

PER SERVING: 129 CALORIES (5% FROM FAT)
FAT 0.7G (SATURATED FAT 0.0G)
PROTEIN 0.8G   CARBOHYDRATE 32.7G
CHOLESTEROL 0MG   SODIUM 2MG

BRUNCH ON THE VERANDA

(pictured on page 36)

Servings		*Calories*
2 crêpes	Crabmeat Crêpes	144
1 cup	Assorted melon balls	56
1 muffin	Lemon-Blueberry Muffins	181
1 cup	Special Mint Tea	76

Serves 8

TOTAL CALORIES PER SERVING: 457
(CALORIES FROM FAT: 17%)

CRABMEAT CRÊPES

Vegetable cooking spray
2 teaspoons reduced-calorie margarine
1⅓ cups sliced fresh mushrooms
1 cup chopped green onions
1 teaspoon dried thyme
1 tablespoon all-purpose flour
1 cup skim milk
1 pound fresh lump crabmeat, drained
2 tablespoons chopped fresh parsley
2 teaspoons lemon juice
¼ teaspoon salt
¼ teaspoon dry mustard
⅛ teaspoon ground red pepper
16 Light Crêpes
Fresh thyme sprigs (optional)

Coat a large nonstick skillet with cooking spray; add margarine. Place over medium-high heat until margarine melts. Add mushrooms, green onions, and 1 teaspoon thyme; sauté 2 to 3 minutes or until vegetables are tender. Reduce heat to low; stir in flour. Cook 1 minute, stirring constantly. Gradually add milk. Cook over medium heat, stirring constantly, until thickened and bubbly. Remove from heat; stir in crabmeat and next 5 ingredients.

Spoon 3 tablespoons crabmeat mixture down center of each of 16 Light Crêpes; roll up crêpes, and place seam side down in two 13- x 9- x 2-inch baking dishes coated with cooking spray. Cover and bake at 350° for 15 to 18 minutes or until

thoroughly heated. Remove cover; broil crêpes 5½ inches from heat (with electric oven door partially opened) 1 minute or until golden. To serve, place 2 crêpes on each serving plate; garnish with thyme sprigs, if desired. Yield: 16 crêpes.

LIGHT CRÊPES

½ cup plus 2 tablespoons all-purpose flour
1⅓ cups skim milk
4 egg whites
Vegetable cooking spray

Combine first 3 ingredients in container of an electric blender or food processor; cover and process 30 seconds. Scrape sides of container; process 30 seconds. Chill batter at least 1 hour.

Coat a 6-inch nonstick crêpe pan or skillet with cooking spray. Place over medium heat just until hot, but not smoking. Pour 2 tablespoons batter into pan; quickly tilt pan in all directions so batter covers bottom of pan in a thin film. Cook 1 minute or until lightly browned.

Lift edge of crêpe to test for doneness. Crêpe is ready for flipping when it can be shaken loose from pan. Flip, and cook about 30 seconds. Place crêpes on a towel to cool. Stack crêpes between layers of wax paper to prevent sticking. Repeat procedure until all batter is used. Yield: 16 (6-inch) crêpes.

PER CRÊPE: 72 CALORIES (16% FROM FAT)
FAT 1.3G (SATURATED FAT 0.2G)
PROTEIN 8.6G   CARBOHYDRATE 6.3G
CHOLESTEROL 29MG   SODIUM 154MG

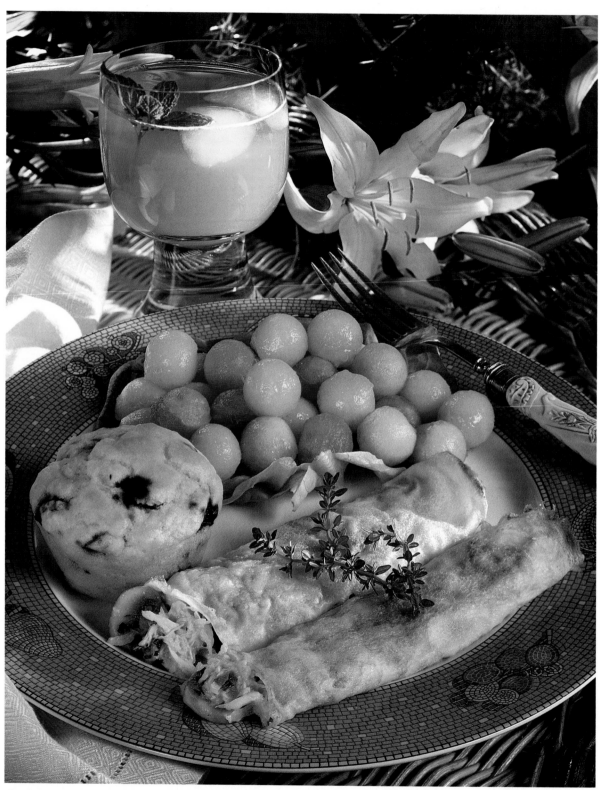

Crabmeat Crêpes (page 35), Lemon-Blueberry Muffins, and Special Mint Tea

LEMON-BLUEBERRY MUFFINS

2 tablespoons sugar
1 tablespoon lemon juice
2½ cups all-purpose flour
2 teaspoons baking powder
½ teaspoon baking soda
¼ teaspoon salt
¼ cup sugar
1½ cups nonfat buttermilk
¼ cup vegetable oil
¼ cup frozen egg substitute, thawed
1 tablespoon grated lemon rind
1 teaspoon vanilla extract
1½ cups frozen unsweetened blueberries,
    thawed
Vegetable cooking spray

Combine 2 tablespoons sugar and lemon juice; stir well, and set aside.

Combine flour and next 4 ingredients in a large bowl, stirring well; make a well in center of flour mixture.

Combine buttermilk, oil, egg substitute, lemon rind, and vanilla; add to flour mixture, stirring just until dry ingredients are moistened. Gently fold in blueberries.

Spoon batter into large (2¾-inch) muffin pans coated with cooking spray, filling three-fourths full. Bake at 375° for 20 minutes.

Remove pans from oven. Brush hot muffins with lemon juice mixture. Bake an additional 6 to 8 minutes or until muffins are golden. Remove muffins from pans immediately, and let cool on wire racks. Yield: 1 dozen.

PER MUFFIN: 181 CALORIES (27% FROM FAT)
FAT 5.4G (SATURATED FAT 0.9G)
PROTEIN 4.2G   CARBOHYDRATE 29.1G
CHOLESTEROL 0MG   SODIUM 142MG

SPECIAL MINT TEA

4 cups water
8 regular-size mint-flavored tea bags
½ cup lemon juice
¼ cup plus 2 tablespoons sugar
2 cups lemon-flavored sparkling mineral
    water, chilled
2 cups unsweetened pineapple juice, chilled
Fresh mint sprigs (optional)

Bring water to a boil; pour over tea bags. Cover and steep 5 minutes. Remove and discard tea bags. Stir in lemon juice and sugar, stirring until sugar dissolves. Cover and chill.

Just before serving, stir in mineral water and pineapple juice. Serve over ice. Garnish each serving with a fresh mint sprig, if desired. Yield: 8 (1-cup) servings.

PER SERVING: 76 CALORIES (1% FROM FAT)
FAT 0.1G (SATURATED FAT 0.0G)
PROTEIN 0.3G   CARBOHYDRATE 19.7G
CHOLESTEROL 0MG   SODIUM 5MG

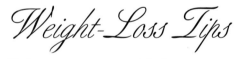

Weight-Loss Tips

Before you start any weight-loss program, ask yourself these questions.

• Is the diet balanced? It takes a variety of foods to provide essential nutrients.

• Does the program fit your lifestyle and budget? If you can't stick to it, forget it.

• Can you splurge occasionally on favorite foods? Moderation is the key.

• Does the plan promote reasonable weight-loss goals? Losing ½ to 1 pound a week is both realistic and healthy.

• Are you encouraged to exercise while dieting? Exercise works in tandem with dieting to produce and maintain weight loss.

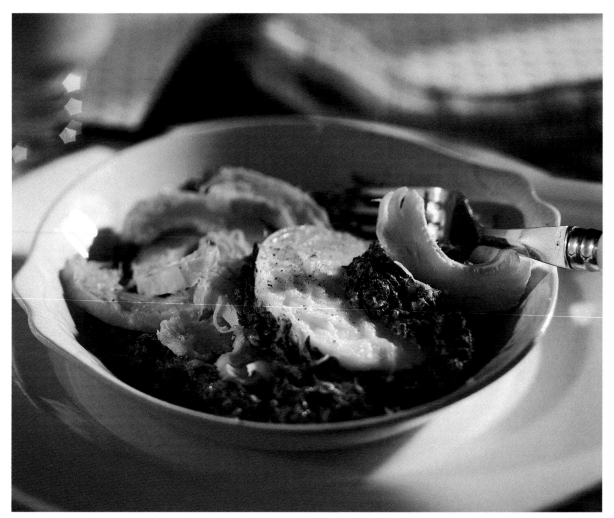

Classic Eggs Sardou

NEW ORLEANS SPECIALTY

Servings		*Calories*
1 serving	Classic Eggs Sardou	232
1 roll	Raspberry-Cheese Buns	145
1 cup	Spicy Vegetable Sipper	47

Serves 2
TOTAL CALORIES PER SERVING: 424
(CALORIES FROM FAT: 25%)

CLASSIC EGGS SARDOU

This famous egg dish is topped with a Parmesan-flavored low-fat cream sauce instead of rich hollandaise.

1 tablespoon all-purpose flour
¾ cup 1% low-fat milk
⅓ cup nonfat sour cream
2 tablespoons grated Parmesan cheese
¼ teaspoon salt
⅛ teaspoon pepper
1 (10-ounce) package frozen chopped spinach, thawed, drained, and squeezed dry
2 eggs
Vegetable cooking spray
2 canned artichoke bottoms, thinly sliced crosswise
2 teaspoons grated Parmesan cheese

Place flour in a saucepan. Gradually add milk, stirring with a wire whisk until blended. Add sour cream, 2 tablespoons Parmesan cheese, salt, pepper, and spinach; stir well. Place over medium heat; cook 8 minutes or until thickened, stirring occasionally. Set aside, and keep warm.

Add water to a large skillet, filling two-thirds full. Bring to a boil; reduce heat, and simmer. Break eggs into each of 2 (6-ounce) custard cups coated with cooking spray. Place custard cups in simmering water in skillet; cover skillet, and cook 6 minutes. Remove custard cups from water; set aside.

Spoon ½ cup spinach mixture onto each of 2 individual plates; fan sliced artichoke bottoms over spinach mixture. Invert poached eggs onto artichokes, and top each egg with ¼ cup spinach mixture. Sprinkle each with 1 teaspoon Parmesan cheese. Broil 5½ inches from heat (with electric oven door partially opened) 3 minutes or until thoroughly heated. Yield: 2 servings.

PER SERVING: 232 CALORIES (32% FROM FAT)
FAT 8.3G (SATURATED FAT 3.2G)
PROTEIN 19.4G   CARBOHYDRATE 20.7G
CHOLESTEROL 220MG   SODIUM 655MG

RASPBERRY-CHEESE BUNS

1 (7-ounce) can refrigerated breadstick dough
1 tablespoon plus 2 teaspoons reduced-fat cream cheese, softened
2 tablespoons seedless raspberry jam
1 teaspoon sugar
Vegetable cooking spray

Unroll dough (do not separate into strips). Spread cream cheese evenly over dough; spread jam evenly over cheese, and sprinkle with sugar. Beginning at short side, tightly roll up dough, jellyroll fashion; pinch seam to seal (do not seal ends of roll).

Cut roll along perforations in dough into 5 slices. Place slices, cut sides up, in muffin pans coated with cooking spray. Bake at 400° for 15 minutes. Yield: 5 rolls.

Note: To reheat leftover rolls, microwave at HIGH for 30 seconds, or wrap the rolls in aluminum foil, and bake at 400° for 10 minutes.

PER ROLL: 145 CALORIES (21% FROM FAT)
FAT 3.4G (SATURATED FAT 1.0G)
PROTEIN 3.5G   CARBOHYDRATE 24.4G
CHOLESTEROL 3MG   SODIUM 319MG

SPICY VEGETABLE SIPPER

1¼ cups no-salt-added vegetable juice
¾ cup canned no-salt-added beef broth
1 teaspoon sugar
½ teaspoon low-sodium Worcestershire sauce
Dash of hot sauce
Lemon slices (optional)

Combine first 5 ingredients in a small saucepan; cook over medium heat until thoroughly heated. Pour into individual mugs. Garnish each with a lemon slice, if desired. Serve warm. Yield: 2 cups.

PER SERVING: 47 CALORIES (4% FROM FAT)
FAT 0.2G (SATURATED FAT 0.0G)
PROTEIN 1.7G   CARBOHYDRATE 9.1G
CHOLESTEROL 0MG   SODIUM 38MG

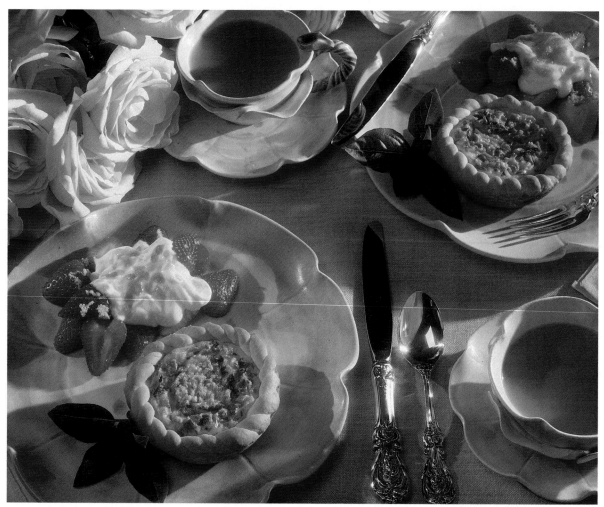

Breakfast in a Bread Basket, Fresh Strawberries with Creamy Yogurt, and Hazelnut Café au Lait

ROMANTIC FRENCH BRUNCH

Servings		*Calories*
1 serving	**Breakfast in a Bread Basket**	269
1 serving	**Fresh Strawberries with Creamy Yogurt**	139
1 cup	**Hazelnut Café au Lait**	45

Serves 2

TOTAL CALORIES PER SERVING: 453
(CALORIES FROM FAT: 16%)

BREAKFAST IN A BREAD BASKET

Vegetable cooking spray
½ cup plus 2 tablespoons low-fat baking mix
2 tablespoons skim milk
3 tablespoons chopped sweet red pepper
3 tablespoons chopped green onions
2 eggs, lightly beaten
1 egg white, lightly beaten
2 tablespoons skim milk
¼ teaspoon garlic powder
¼ teaspoon pepper
Fresh basil sprigs (optional)

Coat 2 (10-ounce) custard cups with cooking spray; set aside. Combine baking mix and 2 tablespoons milk in a small bowl, stirring well. Divide dough into 3 equal portions; shape 2 portions into balls. (Keep remaining portion covered.)

Gently press 1 ball of dough into a 2-inch circle between 2 sheets of heavy-duty plastic wrap. Roll dough, still covered, into a 5-inch circle. Remove top sheet of plastic wrap. Invert and press dough into bottom and 2 inches up sides of prepared custard cup. Remove remaining plastic wrap. Repeat procedure with remaining ball of dough. Divide remaining portion of dough into 4 equal pieces. Roll each piece into a 15-inch rope. Twist 2 ropes together. Repeat procedure with remaining 2 ropes.

Moisten top edge of dough in custard cups with water. Gently press twisted rope around dough in each cup, joining ends of rope together. Set aside.

Coat a small nonstick skillet with cooking spray; place over medium-high heat until hot. Add sweet red pepper and green onions; sauté until tender.

Combine sautéed vegetables, 2 eggs, and next 4 ingredients, stirring well. Pour mixture into pastry shells. Bake at 350° for 35 to 40 minutes or until set. Remove from oven; let stand 5 minutes.

Remove from cups, and garnish with fresh basil sprigs, if desired. Yield: 2 servings.

PER SERVING: 269 CALORIES (20% FROM FAT)
FAT 6.1G (SATURATED FAT 1.7G)
PROTEIN 13.2G CARBOHYDRATE 39.3G
CHOLESTEROL 222MG SODIUM 709MG

FRESH STRAWBERRIES WITH CREAMY YOGURT

1 (8-ounce) carton vanilla low-fat yogurt
1 tablespoon powdered sugar
¼ teaspoon almond extract
1 cup fresh strawberry halves
1 teaspoon brown sugar

Spoon yogurt onto several layers of paper towels; spread to ½-inch thickness. Cover with additional paper towels; let stand 5 minutes. Scrape yogurt into a bowl, using a rubber spatula. Stir in powdered sugar and almond extract. Cover and chill.

Spoon strawberries evenly onto individual plates. Top with yogurt mixture; sprinkle with brown sugar. Yield: 2 servings.

PER SERVING: 139 CALORIES (11% FROM FAT)
FAT 1.7G (SATURATED FAT 0.9G)
PROTEIN 6.0G CARBOHYDRATE 25.8G
CHOLESTEROL 6MG SODIUM 76MG

HAZELNUT CAFÉ AU LAIT

1 cup skim milk
1 teaspoon instant hazelnut-flavored coffee granules
1 cup boiling water

Place milk in a small saucepan, and cook over medium heat until milk is thoroughly heated. (Do not boil.)

Combine coffee granules and water. Pour ½ cup coffee and ½ cup milk into each mug; stir. Serve warm. Yield: 2 (1-cup) servings.

PER SERVING: 45 CALORIES (4% FROM FAT)
FAT 0.2G (SATURATED FAT 0.1G)
PROTEIN 4.3G CARBOHYDRATE 6.4G
CHOLESTEROL 2MG SODIUM 66MG

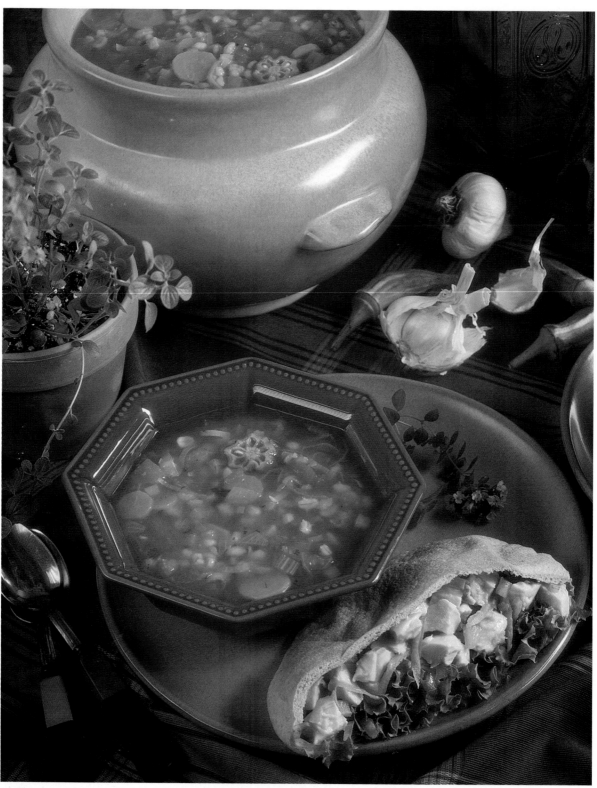

Hearty Vegetable-Barley Soup and Garden Turkey Pocket (menu on page 53)

LUNCHES & LUNCHEONS

"I'll just skip lunch today," you say to yourself. "After all, that's an extra 300 to 400 calories I don't need." But four o'clock arrives, and you're experiencing hunger pangs. At six o'clock, you're at the refrigerator door, and by eight o'clock, you've consumed enough for lunch, supper, and then some!

Instead of binging to battle those hunger pangs, enjoy lunchtime favorites such as a taco salad (page 48) or White Chili and cornbread (page 52). Any of the salads, sandwiches, and soups in this chapter can satisfy your hunger while providing only a moderate number of fat grams. Try the burgers on page 47 or the popular calzones on page 61 for a low-calorie treat.

On those days when you need something really quick for lunch, turn to page 12. You'll find several super-easy lunch ideas complete with fat and calorie information.

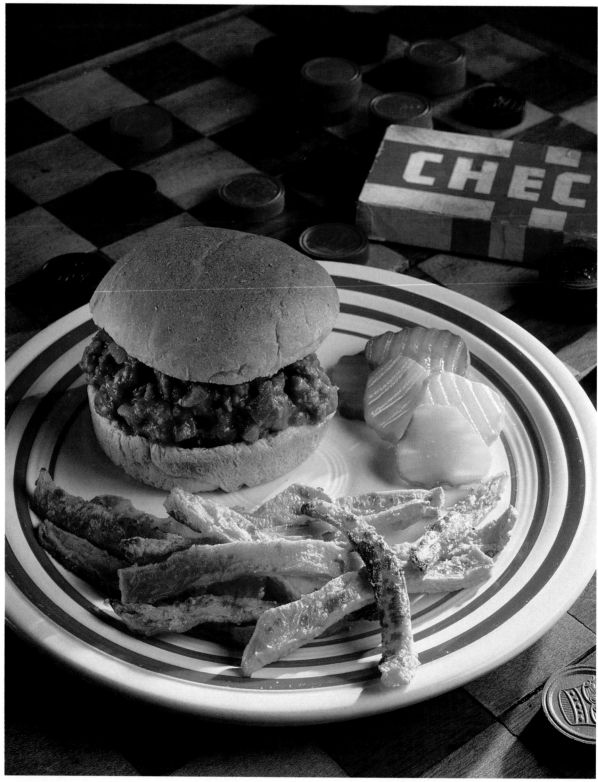

Easy Sloppy Joe and Sweet Potato Sticks

KIDS IN CHARGE

Servings		*Calories*
1 serving	Easy Sloppy Joes	272
1 serving	Sweet Potato Sticks	139
¼ cup	Dill pickles	9

Serves 8
TOTAL CALORIES PER SERVING: 420
(CALORIES FROM FAT: 21%)

EASY SLOPPY JOES

Vegetable cooking spray
1½ pounds ground round
1 cup chopped onion
½ cup chopped green pepper
1 cup ketchup
1 (8-ounce) can no-salt-added tomato sauce
1½ tablespoons low-sodium Worcestershire
    sauce
1½ tablespoons lemon juice
1½ tablespoons prepared mustard
1 tablespoon dark brown sugar
¼ teaspoon garlic powder
¼ teaspoon pepper
8 reduced-calorie whole wheat hamburger
    buns

Coat a large nonstick skillet with cooking spray. Place over medium-high heat until hot. Add ground round, onion, and green pepper. Cook until meat is browned, stirring until it crumbles. Drain and pat dry with paper towels. Wipe drippings from skillet with a paper towel.

Return meat mixture to skillet. Add ketchup and next 7 ingredients; stir well. Cook, uncovered, over medium heat 10 minutes or until thoroughly heated and slightly thickened, stirring frequently.

Spoon meat mixture evenly over bottom halves of buns. Top with remaining bun halves. Yield: 8 servings.

PER SERVING: 272 CALORIES (22% FROM FAT)
FAT 6.7G (SATURATED FAT 2.2G)
PROTEIN 22.1G   CARBOHYDRATE 30.0G
CHOLESTEROL 54MG   SODIUM 673MG

SWEET POTATO STICKS

4 medium-size sweet potatoes (about 2
    pounds), peeled
1 tablespoon vegetable oil
⅓ cup grated Parmesan cheese
Vegetable cooking spray

Cut potatoes lengthwise into ½-inch-thick slices. Cut slices into ¼-inch-wide strips. Place potato strips in a large bowl.

Drizzle oil over potato strips; toss well. Sprinkle with Parmesan cheese, and toss well. Arrange potato strips in a single layer on baking sheets coated with cooking spray.

Bake at 400° for 35 to 40 minutes or until potato strips are crisp and lightly browned, stirring every 10 minutes. Yield: 8 servings.

PER SERVING: 139 CALORIES (20% FROM FAT)
FAT 3.1G (SATURATED FAT 0.9G)
PROTEIN 3.1G   CARBOHYDRATE 25.1G
CHOLESTEROL 3MG   SODIUM 75MG

Healthy Treats

When it comes to nutritious veggies, the sweet potato is one of the best. It's rich in vitamins A and C and provides a healthy dose of fiber. One 4-ounce baked sweet potato contains only 100 calories. Store sweet potatoes in a cool, dark place, not in the refrigerator.

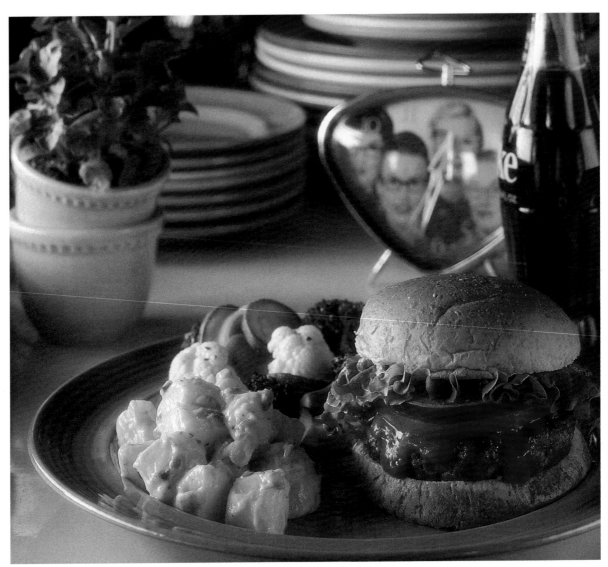

Grilled Mushroom Burger, Creamy Potato Salad, and Cookout Vegetable Packet

BURGERS ON THE GRILL

Servings		*Calories*
1 serving	Grilled Mushroom Burgers	344
1 serving	Creamy Potato Salad	85
1 serving	Cookout Vegetable Packets	56

Serves 6
TOTAL CALORIES PER SERVING: 485
(CALORIES FROM FAT: 22%)

GRILLED MUSHROOM BURGERS

1½ pounds ground round
1½ cups finely chopped fresh mushrooms
¼ cup finely chopped onion
1 tablespoon chili powder
½ teaspoon salt
Vegetable cooking spray
¼ cup plus 2 tablespoons reduced-calorie
     ketchup
6 whole wheat hamburger buns
6 green leaf lettuce leaves
6 tomato slices (¼ inch thick)
6 purple onion slices (¼ inch thick)

Combine first 5 ingredients in a large bowl; stir well. Shape mixture into 6 (½-inch-thick) patties. Coat grill rack with cooking spray; place on grill over medium-hot coals (350° to 400°). Place patties on rack, and grill 5 to 7 minutes on each side or to desired degree of doneness.

Spread 1 tablespoon ketchup over bottom half of each bun; top each with 1 beef patty. Top each patty with a lettuce leaf, tomato slice, onion slice, and top half of bun. Yield: 6 servings.

PER SERVING: 344 CALORIES (29% FROM FAT)
FAT 11.0G (SATURATED FAT 3.6G)
PROTEIN 30.0G   CARBOHYDRATE 30.5G
CHOLESTEROL 87MG   SODIUM 575MG

CREAMY POTATO SALAD

3 cups cooked, peeled, and cubed red potato
2 tablespoons chopped green onions
1 (2-ounce) jar diced pimiento, drained
¼ cup nonfat mayonnaise
¼ cup plain nonfat yogurt
1 tablespoon prepared mustard
1½ teaspoons sugar
1½ teaspoons white wine vinegar
¼ teaspoon salt
¼ teaspoon celery seeds
⅛ teaspoon garlic powder
⅛ teaspoon pepper

Combine potato, green onions, and pimiento in a large bowl, tossing gently to combine.

Combine mayonnaise and next 8 ingredients in a small bowl; stir well. Add mayonnaise mixture to potato mixture; toss gently. Cover and chill thoroughly. Yield: 6 (½-cup) servings.

PER SERVING: 85 CALORIES (3% FROM FAT)
FAT 0.3G (SATURATED FAT 0.0G)
PROTEIN 2.0G   CARBOHYDRATE 19.1G
CHOLESTEROL 0MG   SODIUM 269MG

COOKOUT VEGETABLE PACKETS

1½ cups sliced yellow squash
1½ cups sliced zucchini
1½ cups cauliflower flowerets
1½ cups broccoli flowerets
1 cup thinly sliced carrot
1 medium onion, thinly sliced
⅔ cup commercial oil-free Italian dressing
½ teaspoon dried basil
¼ teaspoon salt
¼ teaspoon pepper
Vegetable cooking spray

Combine first 6 ingredients in a large bowl, tossing gently. Combine Italian dressing, basil, salt, and pepper in a small bowl, stirring well. Pour dressing mixture over vegetable mixture, and toss gently to combine.

Divide vegetable mixture evenly among 6 large squares of heavy-duty aluminum foil. Wrap vegetables securely, sealing edges of foil packets.

Coat grill rack with cooking spray; place on grill over medium-hot coals (350° to 400°). Place vegetable packets on grill rack, and grill 4 to 5 minutes or until vegetables are crisp-tender, turning packets once. Yield: 6 servings.

PER SERVING: 56 CALORIES (5% FROM FAT)
FAT 0.3G (SATURATED FAT 0.1G)
PROTEIN 2.5G   CARBOHYDRATE 12.2G
CHOLESTEROL 0MG   SODIUM 358MG

LUNCHTIME FIESTA
(pictured on page 2)

Servings		Calories
1 serving	Taco Salad for Two	301
1 serving	Mexican Corn	96
1 medium	Kiwifruit	44
1 cup	Iced tea	2

Serves 2
TOTAL CALORIES PER SERVING: 443
(CALORIES FROM FAT: 25%)

TACO SALAD FOR TWO

Lighten the fat and calories in this popular salad by using ground round, reduced-fat cheese, and nonfat sour cream.

2 (8-inch) flour tortillas
Vegetable cooking spray
⅓ pound ground round
½ cup water
2 tablespoons chopped green onions
2 teaspoons chili powder
⅛ teaspoon ground cumin
2 cups shredded iceberg lettuce
1 small tomato, seeded and chopped
2 tablespoons (½ ounce) reduced-fat shredded
    Cheddar cheese
2 tablespoons nonfat sour cream
½ cup commercial no-salt-added salsa

Cut each tortilla into 8 wedges; place on a baking sheet. Bake at 350° for 10 to 12 minutes or until lightly browned. Set aside.

Coat a large nonstick skillet with cooking spray; place over medium-high heat until hot. Add ground round, and cook over medium heat until browned, stirring to crumble meat. Drain and pat dry with paper towels. Wipe drippings from skillet with a paper towel. Return meat to skillet; add water, green onions, chili powder, and cumin, stirring well to combine. Bring meat mixture to a boil; reduce heat, and simmer 10 minutes.

For each salad, layer half of tortilla wedges, lettuce, meat mixture, and chopped tomato on each of 2 serving plates. Top each salad with 1 tablespoon shredded Cheddar cheese and 1 tablespoon sour cream. Serve with salsa. Yield: 2 servings.

PER SERVING: 301 CALORIES (28% FROM FAT)
FAT 9.5G (SATURATED FAT 2.9G)
PROTEIN 24.3G CARBOHYDRATE 29.5G
CHOLESTEROL 50MG SODIUM 443MG

MEXICAN CORN

Vegetable cooking spray
1 teaspoon margarine
1 cup frozen yellow corn, thawed
3 tablespoons water
2 tablespoons chopped green pepper
2 tablespoons chopped sweet red pepper
2 tablespoons chopped purple onion
1 tablespoon chopped fresh cilantro
⅛ teaspoon salt

Coat a medium nonstick skillet with cooking spray; add margarine. Place over medium-high heat until hot. Add corn and remaining 6 ingredients; cook over medium heat 5 minutes or until tender, stirring occasionally. Yield: 2 (½-cup) servings.

PER SERVING: 96 CALORIES (23% FROM FAT)
FAT 2.4G (SATURATED FAT 0.4G)
PROTEIN 2.8G CARBOHYDRATE 18.9G
CHOLESTEROL 0MG SODIUM 175MG

CHICKEN SALAD WITH A TWIST

Servings		Calories
1 serving	Southwestern Chicken Salad Sandwiches	225
1 serving	Vegetable Coleslaw	75
1 medium	Fresh apple	81

Serves 4

TOTAL CALORIES PER SERVING: 381
(CALORIES FROM FAT: 17%)

SOUTHWESTERN CHICKEN SALAD SANDWICHES

This chicken salad is much lower in fat than the traditional version. Salsa, cumin, and ground red pepper give it a spicy flavor.

4 ounces nonfat cream cheese, softened
⅓ cup nonfat sour cream
2 tablespoons no-salt-added mild salsa
½ teaspoon ground cumin
¼ teaspoon salt
¼ teaspoon ground red pepper
1½ cups shredded cooked chicken
⅓ cup finely chopped sweet red pepper
⅓ cup minced green onions
8 (¾-ounce) slices reduced-calorie whole wheat bread, toasted
16 medium-size fresh spinach leaves
1 cup alfalfa sprouts

Combine first 6 ingredients in a small bowl. Stir in chicken, sweet red pepper, and green onions. Spread mixture evenly over 4 slices of bread; top evenly with spinach leaves. Place alfalfa sprouts evenly over spinach; top with remaining 4 bread slices. Yield: 4 servings.

PER SERVING: 225 CALORIES (24% FROM FAT)
FAT 6.0G (SATURATED FAT 1.4G)
PROTEIN 25.3G CARBOHYDRATE 17.6G
CHOLESTEROL 52MG SODIUM 595MG

VEGETABLE COLESLAW

Make lunchtime easier by preparing this slaw a day ahead and chilling it overnight.

1½ cups shredded red cabbage
1 cup shredded carrot
¾ cup shredded yellow squash
¾ cup shredded zucchini
½ cup chopped green pepper
⅓ cup finely chopped onion
¼ cup unsweetened pineapple juice
1½ tablespoons sugar
3 tablespoons cider vinegar
2 tablespoons water
½ teaspoon chicken-flavored bouillon granules
¼ teaspoon paprika
¼ teaspoon celery seeds
⅛ teaspoon garlic powder
Dash of ground red pepper

Combine first 6 ingredients in a large bowl. Combine pineapple juice and next 8 ingredients in a bowl, stirring well. Pour over vegetable mixture; toss gently. Cover and chill at least 4 hours. Yield: 4 (1-cup) servings.

PER SERVING: 75 CALORIES (7% FROM FAT)
FAT 0.6G (SATURATED FAT 0.1G)
PROTEIN 2.0G CARBOHYDRATE 17.7G
CHOLESTEROL 0MG SODIUM 118MG

PICNIC IN THE PARK

Servings		*Calories*
1 serving	Chicken and Black-Eyed Pea Salad	220
1 serving	Gingered Melon Balls	62
1 wedge	Sweet Onion Focaccia	124

Serves 6

TOTAL CALORIES PER SERVING: 406
(CALORIES FROM FAT: 15%)

CHICKEN AND BLACK-EYED PEA SALAD

2 (15.8-ounce) cans black-eyed peas, drained
2 cups chopped cooked chicken breast
¾ cup minced celery
¾ cup minced sweet red pepper
½ cup minced green onions
⅓ cup minced fresh cilantro
3 tablespoons commercial oil-free Italian
    dressing
2 tablespoons country-style Dijon mustard
6 red leaf lettuce leaves

Combine first 8 ingredients in a large bowl; stir well. Cover and chill.

To serve, place a lettuce leaf on each of 6 individual salad plates; spoon 1 cup black-eyed pea mixture onto each lettuce leaf. Yield: 6 servings.

PER SERVING: 220 CALORIES (13% FROM FAT)
FAT 3.1G (SATURATED FAT 0.7G)
PROTEIN 24.2G   CARBOHYDRATE 23.8G
CHOLESTEROL 40MG   SODIUM 471MG

GINGERED MELON BALLS

¾ cup water
¼ cup sugar
1 teaspoon peeled, grated gingerroot
1 cup cantaloupe balls
1 cup honeydew melon balls
1 cup watermelon balls

Combine water, sugar, and gingerroot in a medium saucepan. Bring to a boil; reduce heat, and simmer, uncovered, 14 minutes, stirring occasionally. Remove from heat, and let cool completely.

Combine melon balls in a medium bowl. Pour sugar mixture over melon balls, and toss gently. Cover and chill. Yield: 6 (½-cup) servings.

PER SERVING: 62 CALORIES (3% FROM FAT)
FAT 0.2G (SATURATED FAT 0.1G)
PROTEIN 0.6G   CARBOHYDRATE 15.6G
CHOLESTEROL 0MG   SODIUM 7MG

SWEET ONION FOCACCIA

1 tablespoon cumin seeds
1 tablespoon reduced-calorie margarine
1½ cups finely chopped onion
1 teaspoon sugar
2 cups plus 2 tablespoons bread flour, divided
½ cup whole wheat flour
½ teaspoon salt
1 package active dry yeast
1 cup warm skim milk (120° to 130°)
3 tablespoons olive oil
2 tablespoons bread flour
Vegetable cooking spray

Place cumin seeds in a large nonstick skillet; cook over medium-high heat until toasted, stirring frequently. Remove from skillet, and cool. Add margarine to skillet; place over medium heat until margarine melts. Add onion and sugar; sauté until onion is browned. Set aside.

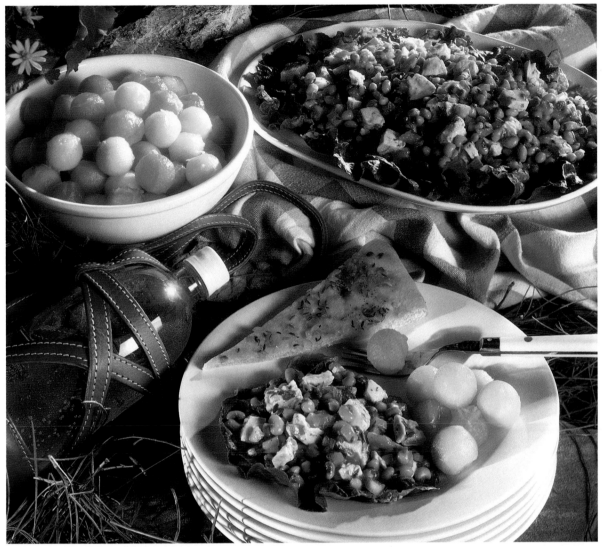

Chicken and Black-Eyed Pea Salad, Gingered Melon Balls, and Sweet Onion Focaccia

Combine 1 cup bread flour, whole wheat flour, salt, and yeast in a large mixing bowl; stir well. Add milk and olive oil to flour mixture, beating well at low speed of an electric mixer. Beat an additional 2 minutes at medium speed. Gradually stir in enough of the remaining 1 cup plus 2 tablespoons bread flour to make a soft dough.

Sprinkle 2 tablespoons bread flour over work surface. Turn dough out onto surface; knead until smooth and elastic (8 to 10 minutes). Place in a large bowl coated with cooking spray, turning to coat top. Cover; let rise in a warm place (85°), free from drafts, 45 to 55 minutes or until doubled in bulk.

Punch dough down. Press onto a 15-inch round pizza pan coated with cooking spray. Poke holes in dough at 1-inch intervals with handle of a wooden spoon. Spread onion mixture over dough; press lightly. Sprinkle with toasted cumin seeds. Let rise, uncovered, in a warm place, free from drafts, 30 minutes. Bake at 375° for 20 minutes or until golden. Cut into 16 wedges. Serve warm or at room temperature. Yield: 16 servings.

PER WEDGE: 124 CALORIES (26% FROM FAT)
FAT 3.6G (SATURATED FAT 0.4G)
PROTEIN 3.7G   CARBOHYDRATE 19.3G
CHOLESTEROL 0MG   SODIUM 90MG

COLD-WEATHER LUNCH

Servings		_Calories_
1 cup	White Chili	173
1 square	Light Cornbread Squares	161
1 cup	Skim milk	86

Serves 9

TOTAL CALORIES PER SERVING: 420
(CALORIES FROM FAT: 17%)

WHITE CHILI

Vegetable cooking spray
1 tablespoon olive oil
1 pound skinned, boned chicken breasts, diced
½ cup chopped shallots
3 cloves garlic, minced
1 (18-ounce) can tomatillos, drained and
   coarsely chopped
1 (14½-ounce) can no-salt-added whole
   tomatoes, undrained and coarsely chopped
1 (13¾-ounce) can no-salt-added chicken broth
1 (4-ounce) can chopped green chile peppers,
   undrained
½ teaspoon dried oregano
½ teaspoon coriander seeds, crushed
¼ teaspoon ground cumin
2 (15½-ounce) cans cannellini beans or other
   white beans, rinsed and drained
3 tablespoons fresh lime juice
¼ teaspoon pepper
¼ cup plus 2 tablespoons (1½ ounces)
   shredded reduced-fat sharp Cheddar
   cheese

  Coat a large saucepan with cooking spray; add olive oil, and place over medium-high heat until hot. Add diced chicken breast, and sauté 3 minutes or until chicken is done. Remove chicken from pan, and set aside.
  Add shallots and garlic to pan, and sauté until tender. Stir in tomatillos and next 6 ingredients. Bring to a boil; reduce heat, and simmer 20 minutes. Add chicken and beans; cook 5 minutes or until thoroughly heated. Stir in lime juice and pepper.

Ladle chili into serving bowls, and top with cheese. Yield: 9 (1-cup) servings.

PER SERVING: 173 CALORIES (20% FROM FAT)
FAT 3.8G (SATURATED FAT 0.9G)
PROTEIN 17.2G   CARBOHYDRATE 16.6G
CHOLESTEROL 32MG   SODIUM 583MG

LIGHT CORNBREAD SQUARES

1½ cups yellow cornmeal
½ cup all-purpose flour
1 teaspoon baking powder
1 teaspoon baking soda
¼ teaspoon salt
2 teaspoons sugar
1⅔ cups nonfat buttermilk
¼ cup frozen egg substitute, thawed
2 tablespoons vegetable oil
Vegetable cooking spray

  Combine first 6 ingredients in a large bowl; make a well in center of mixture. Combine buttermilk, egg substitute, and oil; add to dry ingredients, stirring just until dry ingredients are moistened.
  Pour batter into an 8-inch square pan coated with cooking spray. Bake at 400° for 22 to 25 minutes or until golden. Cut into squares. Yield: 9 servings.

PER SQUARE: 161 CALORIES (21% FROM FAT)
FAT 3.7G (SATURATED FAT 0.7G)
PROTEIN 5.0G   CARBOHYDRATE 26.7G
CHOLESTEROL 2MG   SODIUM 250MG

SOUP AND SANDWICH COMBO

(pictured on page 42)

<u>Servings</u>		<u>Calories</u>
1½ cups	Hearty Vegetable-Barley Soup	113
1 serving	Garden Turkey Pockets	184
½ cup	Seedless red grapes	57

Serves 4

TOTAL CALORIES PER SERVING: 354
(CALORIES FROM FAT: 9%)

HEARTY VEGETABLE-BARLEY SOUP

This soup is even better the second time around. Refrigerating the leftovers for a day or two lets the flavors blend and intensify.

Vegetable cooking spray
1 cup chopped onion
½ cup chopped celery
2 tablespoons chopped fresh parsley
1 clove garlic, minced
4 (13¾-ounce) cans no-salt-added beef broth, undiluted
2 (14½-ounce) cans no-salt-added whole tomatoes, undrained and chopped
1 cup thinly sliced carrot
½ cup pearl barley, uncooked
½ teaspoon salt
¼ teaspoon pepper
¼ teaspoon dried oregano
¼ teaspoon dried basil
¼ teaspoon dried thyme
1 bay leaf
1 cup thinly sliced leeks
1 cup sliced fresh okra
½ cup peeled, diced turnips

Coat a large Dutch oven with cooking spray; place over medium-high heat until hot. Add onion, and next 3 ingredients; sauté 4 minutes. Add broth and next 9 ingredients to vegetable mixture; bring to a boil, stirring occasionally. Cover, reduce heat, and simmer 20 minutes, stirring occasionally.

Add leeks, okra, and turnips to broth mixture; stir. Cover and simmer 15 to 20 minutes or until vegetables are tender, stirring occasionally. Remove and discard bay leaf. Yield: 8 (1½-cup) servings.

PER SERVING: 113 CALORIES (3% FROM FAT)
FAT 0.4G (SATURATED FAT 0.1G)
PROTEIN 3.5G CARBOHYDRATE 23.0G
CHOLESTEROL 0MG SODIUM 190MG

GARDEN TURKEY POCKETS

1½ cups cubed cooked turkey breast
½ cup coarsely shredded carrot
½ cup diced celery
2½ tablespoons plain nonfat yogurt
2 tablespoons commercial oil-free Italian dressing
2 (6-inch) whole wheat pita bread rounds, cut in half crosswise
Green leaf lettuce leaves (optional)

Combine first 5 ingredients; stir. Cover and chill. Line pita halves with lettuce, if desired. Spoon ½ cup turkey mixture into each half. Yield: 4 servings.

PER SERVING: 184 CALORIES (13% FROM FAT)
FAT 2.6G (SATURATED FAT 0.6G)
PROTEIN 19.8G CARBOHYDRATE 17.5G
CHOLESTEROL 48MG SODIUM 148MG

LUNCH BOX FAVORITES

Servings		_Calories_
1 serving	Turkey Sandwiches	270
1 serving	Carrot-Raisin Salad	166
1 cookie	Molasses Crinkles	48

Serves 4

TOTAL CALORIES PER SERVING: 484
(CALORIES FROM FAT: 16%)

TURKEY SANDWICHES

¼ cup nonfat cream cheese
¼ cup seedless raspberry jam
1 tablespoon chopped walnuts, toasted
8 (¾-ounce) slices whole wheat bread
4 curly leaf lettuce leaves
½ pound thinly sliced cooked turkey breast

Combine first 3 ingredients in a small bowl; stir well. Spread 2 tablespoons cream cheese mixture over each of 4 slices of bread. Top each with 1 lettuce leaf, 2 ounces turkey, and remaining bread slices. Yield: 4 servings.

PER SERVING: 270 CALORIES (14% FROM FAT)
FAT 4.3G (SATURATED FAT 0.9G)
PROTEIN 24.1G CARBOHYDRATE 34.7G
CHOLESTEROL 43MG SODIUM 354MG

CARROT-RAISIN SALAD

4 cups coarsely shredded carrot
½ cup raisins
3 tablespoons reduced-calorie mayonnaise
1 (8-ounce) can unsweetened crushed
    pineapple, undrained

Combine all ingredients in a bowl; toss well. Cover and chill 1 hour. Yield: 4 (1-cup) servings.

PER SERVING: 166 CALORIES (18% FROM FAT)
FAT 3.3G (SATURATED FAT 0.4G)
PROTEIN 2.0G CARBOHYDRATE 35.1G
CHOLESTEROL 4MG SODIUM 125MG

MOLASSES CRINKLES

¼ cup margarine, softened
¾ cup plus 1½ tablespoons sugar, divided
¼ cup molasses
1 egg
2 cups all-purpose flour
2 teaspoons baking soda
¼ teaspoon salt
1¾ teaspoons ground cinnamon, divided
Vegetable cooking spray

Beat margarine at medium speed of an electric mixer until creamy; gradually add ¾ cup sugar, beating well. Add molasses and egg; beat well.

Combine flour, baking soda, salt, and 1½ teaspoons ground cinnamon in a small bowl, stirring well. Gradually add flour mixture to margarine mixture, beating until blended. Cover dough, and chill 1 hour.

Combine remaining 1½ tablespoons sugar and remaining ¼ teaspoon ground cinnamon in a small bowl, and set aside.

Shape dough into 48 (1-inch) balls; roll balls in sugar mixture. Place balls, 2 inches apart, on cookie sheets coated with cooking spray. Bake at 350° for 8 minutes or until golden. Cool slightly on cookie sheets. Remove from cookie sheets, and cool completely on wire racks. Yield: 4 dozen.

PER COOKIE: 48 CALORIES (21% FROM FAT)
FAT 1.1G (SATURATED FAT 0.2G)
PROTEIN 0.7G CARBOHYDRATE 8.7G
CHOLESTEROL 5MG SODIUM 78MG

DELI-STYLE LUNCH

Servings		*Calories*
1 serving	Grilled New Yorker	276
1¼ cups	Spiced Tomato Soup	164
1 cup	Sparkling mineral water	0

Serves 2
TOTAL CALORIES PER SERVING: 440
(CALORIES FROM FAT: 14%)

GRILLED NEW YORKER

1 tablespoon reduced-calorie mayonnaise
1 teaspoon Dijon mustard
4 (1-ounce) slices rye bread
2 (¾-ounce) slices Swiss-flavored nonfat
　　process cheese
4 ounces thinly sliced lean, lower-salt smoked ham
1 cup thinly sliced green cabbage
Vegetable cooking spray

　Combine mayonnaise and mustard in a bowl; stir.
Spread mixture over each of 2 bread slices; top each
with 1 cheese slice, 1 ounce ham, ½ cup cabbage,
and 1 ounce ham. Top with remaining bread slices.
　Coat a nonstick skillet with cooking spray; place
over medium heat until hot. Cook sandwiches 3
minutes on each side or until golden. Yield: 2 servings.

PER SERVING: 276 CALORIES (20% FROM FAT)
FAT 6.0G (SATURATED FAT 2.0G)
PROTEIN 20.4G CARBOHYDRATE 36.2G
CHOLESTEROL 35MG SODIUM 1183MG

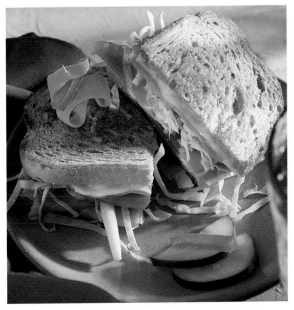

Grilled New Yorker

SPICED TOMATO SOUP

Vegetable cooking spray
¾ cup peeled, chopped sweet potato
¼ cup chopped shallots
2 cloves garlic, minced
2 tablespoons sun-dried tomato tidbits
¼ teaspoon chili powder
1 (14½-ounce) can no-salt-added stewed tomatoes
1 (5½-ounce) can spicy-hot vegetable juice

　Coat a medium saucepan with cooking spray, and
place over medium-high heat until hot. Add sweet
potato, shallots, and garlic, and sauté 4 minutes.
Add sun-dried tomato bits and remaining ingredients, and bring to a boil. Cover, reduce heat, and
simmer 40 minutes or until sweet potato is tender.
　Place ¾ cup of tomato mixture in container of an
electric blender; cover and process until smooth.
Add tomato puree to mixture in pan; stir well.
Yield: 2 (1¼-cup) servings.

PER SERVING: 164 CALORIES (4% FROM FAT)
FAT 0.8G (SATURATED FAT 0.1G)
PROTEIN 5.0G CARBOHYDRATE 36.7G
CHOLESTEROL 0MG SODIUM 162MG

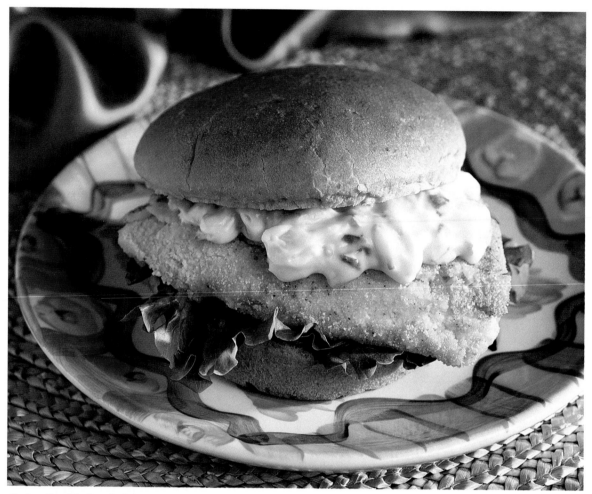

Spicy Catfish Sandwich

FISH-ON-A-BUN

<u>Servings</u>		<u>Calories</u>
1 serving	Spicy Catfish Sandwiches	301
1 serving	Cucumber and Onion Salad	42
1 serving	Fresh Fruit with Mango Sauce	70
1 cup	Iced tea	2

Serves 4

TOTAL CALORIES PER SERVING: 415
(CALORIES FROM FAT: 18%)

SPICY CATFISH SANDWICHES

The fat-free tartar sauce also complements grilled fish or chicken.

4 (4-ounce) farm-raised catfish fillets
¼ cup hot sauce
¾ cup cornmeal
⅛ teaspoon salt
Butter-flavored vegetable cooking spray
2 teaspoons reduced-calorie margarine
4 green leaf lettuce leaves
4 reduced-calorie whole wheat hamburger
      buns
Tropical Tartar Sauce

Place fillets in a shallow dish; pour hot sauce over fillets, turning to coat. Cover and marinate in refrigerator 30 minutes.

Combine cornmeal and salt in a container; dredge fillets in cornmeal mixture, shaking off excess.

Coat a large nonstick skillet with cooking spray; add margarine. Place over medium-high heat until margarine melts. Add fillets, and cook 3 to 4 minutes on each side or until fish flakes easily when tested with a fork.

Place a lettuce leaf on bottom half of each bun; top each with a fillet. Spoon 2 tablespoons Tropical Tartar Sauce over each fillet; top with remaining bun halves. Yield: 4 servings.

TROPICAL TARTAR SAUCE
2 tablespoons nonfat mayonnaise
2 tablespoons nonfat sour cream
1 tablespoon crushed unsweetened pineapple,
      undrained
2 teaspoons diced pimiento
2 teaspoons minced green onions
2 teaspoons finely chopped sweet pickle

Combine all ingredients in a small bowl, stirring well. Cover and chill thoroughly. Yield: ½ cup.

PER SERVING: 301 CALORIES (23% FROM FAT)
FAT 7.6G (SATURATED FAT 1.5G)
PROTEIN 24.7G CARBOHYDRATE 31.4G
CHOLESTEROL 66MG SODIUM 537MG

CUCUMBER AND ONION SALAD

4 cups thinly sliced, unpeeled cucumber
1 cup thinly sliced onion
½ teaspoon salt
⅓ cup nonfat sour cream
2 tablespoons rice wine vinegar
1 teaspoon dried dillweed
½ cup thinly sliced radishes

Combine first 3 ingredients in a bowl. Let stand 30 minutes. Drain and pat dry with paper towels.

Combine sour cream, vinegar, and dillweed in a bowl, stirring until smooth. Add cucumber mixture and radishes; toss gently. Cover and chill 1 hour. Yield: 4 (1-cup) servings.

PER SERVING: 42 CALORIES (6% FROM FAT)
FAT 0.3G (SATURATED FAT 0.0G)
PROTEIN 2.4G CARBOHYDRATE 7.9G
CHOLESTEROL 0MG SODIUM 167MG

FRESH FRUIT WITH MANGO SAUCE

1 cup peeled, cubed fresh mango
1½ teaspoons fresh lime juice
2 cups fresh pineapple chunks
1 cup sliced fresh strawberries

Position knife blade in food processor bowl; add cubed mango, and process until smooth. Combine mango puree and lime juice in a bowl, and stir well. Cover and chill.

To serve, spoon ½ cup pineapple chunks into each of 4 dessert compotes, and top with ¼ cup sliced strawberries and 2 tablespoons of mango mixture. Yield: 4 servings.

PER SERVING: 70 CALORIES (8% FROM FAT)
FAT 0.6G (SATURATED FAT 0.1G)
PROTEIN 0.7G CARBOHYDRATE 17.8G
CHOLESTEROL 0MG SODIUM 2MG

A Different Tuna Sandwich

Servings		*Calories*
1 serving	Tuna Burgers	335
8 wedges	Roasted potato wedges	129
1 cup	Assorted raw vegetables	38

Serves 4
TOTAL CALORIES PER SERVING: 502
(CALORIES FROM FAT: 18%)

Tuna Burgers

2 tablespoons nonfat mayonnaise
2 tablespoons creamy mustard-mayonnaise
   blend
1 egg white
2 (6⅛-ounce) cans albacore tuna in water,
   drained and flaked
½ cup dry breadcrumbs, divided
¼ cup chopped green onions
Vegetable cooking spray
¼ cup nonfat mayonnaise
4 (1½-ounce) hamburger buns, split
4 lettuce leaves
4 slices tomato
4 slices sweet onion

Combine first 3 ingredients in a bowl; stir well.
Add tuna, ¼ cup breadcrumbs, and green onions;
stir well. Divide mixture into 4 equal portions,
shaping each into a 4-inch patty. Press remaining
breadcrumbs evenly onto both sides of patties.

Coat a large nonstick skillet with cooking spray;
place skillet over medium-high heat until hot. Add
patties; cover and cook patties 3 minutes. Carefully
turn patties, and cook, uncovered, 3 minutes or
until patties are golden.

Spread mayonnaise evenly on the bun tops and
bottoms. Place lettuce, tomato, onion, and patties
on bottom halves of buns; place tops on sandwiches.
Yield: 4 servings.

PER SERVING: 335 CALORIES (20% FROM FAT)
FAT 7.6G (SATURATED FAT 1.2G)
PROTEIN 23.5G CARBOHYDRATE 41.8G
CHOLESTEROL 41MG SODIUM 869MG

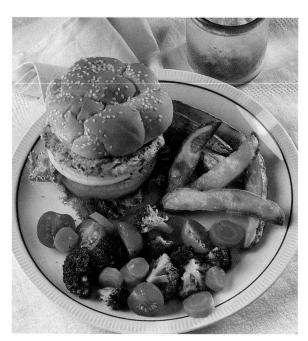

Tuna Burger

Menu Helper

To roast potatoes, cut into thin wedges, and
arrange in a single layer on a baking sheet
coated with vegetable cooking spray. Coat cut
potatoes with butter-flavored, olive oil-flavored,
or plain vegetable cooking spray. Bake at 400°
for 30 minutes or until tender.

HEALTHY SALAD LUNCH

Servings		*Calories*
1 serving	White Bean-Vegetable Salad	278
1 cup	Tomato soup	85
4 crackers	Saltine crackers	51
1 serving	Blueberries with Yogurt Topping	81

Serves 4

TOTAL CALORIES PER SERVING: 495
(CALORIES FROM FAT: 21%)

WHITE BEAN-VEGETABLE SALAD

¼ cup water
¾ cup diced carrot
3 tablespoons red wine vinegar
2 tablespoons olive oil
¼ teaspoon salt
¼ teaspoon dried basil
⅛ teaspoon dried thyme
⅛ teaspoon dried crushed red pepper
⅛ teaspoon rubbed sage
⅛ teaspoon black pepper
2 cloves garlic, minced
1 cup diced sweet yellow pepper
½ cup thinly sliced green onions
10 cherry tomatoes, quartered
2 (16-ounce) cans cannellini beans or other
   white beans, rinsed and drained
4 cups torn curly endive

Bring ¼ cup water to a boil in a small saucepan; add carrot, and cook 1 minute. Drain; set aside.

Combine vinegar and next 8 ingredients in a large bowl, and stir well with a wire whisk. Add carrot, yellow pepper, green onions, tomatoes, and beans, and toss well. For each serving, place 1 cup endive on a salad plate, and top with 1½ cups bean mixture. Yield: 4 servings.

PER SERVING: 278 CALORIES (26% FROM FAT)
FAT 7.9G (SATURATED FAT 1.1G)
PROTEIN 13.5G CARBOHYDRATE 40.0G
CHOLESTEROL 0MG SODIUM 499MG

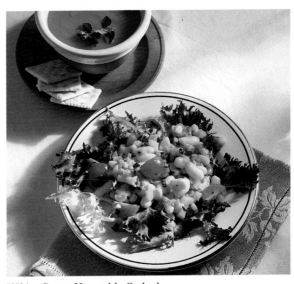

White Bean-Vegetable Salad

BLUEBERRIES WITH YOGURT TOPPING

2 cups fresh blueberries
½ cup lemon low-fat yogurt
Fresh mint sprigs (optional)

Divide blueberries among 4 dessert dishes; top each with 2 tablespoons yogurt. Garnish with mint, if desired. Yield: 4 servings.

PER SERVING: 81 CALORIES (6% FROM FAT)
FAT 0.5G (SATURATED FAT 0.0G)
PROTEIN 1.6G CARBOHYDRATE 18.8G
CHOLESTEROL 0MG SODIUM 24MG

GREEK-STYLE PIZZAS

Servings		*Calories*
1 serving	Mediterranean Pita Rounds	379
1 cup	Green salad with nonfat salad dressing	16

Serves 8
TOTAL CALORIES PER SERVING: 395
(CALORIES FROM FAT: 15%)

MEDITERRANEAN PITA ROUNDS

2 (15-ounce) cans no-salt-added garbanzo
　　beans, drained
¼ cup skim milk
¼ cup fresh lemon juice
5 cloves garlic
8 (8-inch) pita bread rounds
1 teaspoon olive oil
1 (10-ounce) package frozen chopped spinach,
　　thawed and drained
2 cups chopped tomato
1 cup diced green pepper
1 cup diced sweet red pepper
½ cup crumbled feta cheese
⅓ cup sliced ripe olives

Position knife blade in food processor bowl; add first 4 ingredients. Process until smooth, scraping sides of processor bowl occasionally. Set aside.

Arrange pita bread rounds on ungreased baking sheets; brush with olive oil. Bake at 450° for 6 minutes. Spread bean mixture evenly over pitas, leaving a ½-inch border. Arrange remaining ingredients evenly over pita rounds. Bake at 450° for 5 minutes or until thoroughly heated and crust is crisp. Yield: 8 servings.

PER SERVING: 379 CALORIES (16% FROM FAT)
FAT 6.6G (SATURATED FAT 1.7G)
PROTEIN 13.5G　CARBOHYDRATE 64.8G
CHOLESTEROL 6MG　SODIUM 602MG

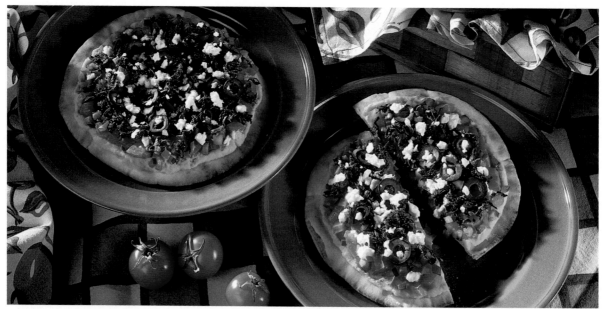

Mediterranean Pita Rounds

A HIKER'S DELIGHT

Servings		Calories
1 serving	Roasted Vegetable and Feta Calzones	313
½ cup	Celery sticks	10
4 cookies	Granola Meringue Cookies	48

Serves 8
TOTAL CALORIES PER SERVING: 371
(CALORIES FROM FAT: 21%)

ROASTED VEGETABLE AND FETA CALZONES

3 cups diced peeled eggplant
2 cups chopped yellow onion
1½ cups diced mushroom
1½ cups diced zucchini
1 cup diced sweet red pepper
1 tablespoon olive oil
½ teaspoon pepper
¼ teaspoon salt
1 cup (4 ounces) crumbled feta cheese
½ cup chopped fresh basil
1 (1-pound) loaf frozen white bread dough, thawed
Vegetable cooking spray
1 egg white
1 tablespoon water

Combine eggplant and next 7 ingredients on a 15- x 10- x 1-inch jellyroll pan; stir well, and spread evenly. Bake at 425° for 45 minutes, stirring every 15 minutes. Spoon vegetables into a bowl; stir in cheese and basil.

Divide dough into 8 equal portions. Working with 1 portion at a time (cover remaining dough to keep from drying out), roll each portion into a 7-inch circle on a lightly floured surface. Spoon ½ cup vegetable mixture onto half of each circle; moisten edges of dough with water. Fold dough over filling; press edges together with a fork. Place calzones on a baking sheet coated with cooking spray.

Combine egg white and 1 tablespoon water; brush over calzones. Bake at 375° for 20 minutes or until golden. Let cool on a wire rack. Serve warm or at room temperature. Yield: 8 servings.

PER SERVING: 313 CALORIES (23% FROM FAT)
FAT 8.0G (SATURATED FAT 3.1G)
PROTEIN 11.7G CARBOHYDRATE 49.5G
CHOLESTEROL 13MG SODIUM 683MG

GRANOLA MERINGUE COOKIES

3 egg whites
½ teaspoon cream of tartar
¼ cup plus 2 tablespoons sugar
¾ cup low-fat granola cereal without raisins
¼ teaspoon vanilla extract
¼ teaspoon almond extract

Line 2 large baking sheets with parchment or heavy brown paper; set aside. Beat egg whites and cream of tartar at high speed of an electric mixer until foamy. Gradually add sugar, 1 tablespoon at a time, beating until stiff peaks form and sugar dissolves (2 to 4 minutes). Fold in cereal and flavorings.

Drop egg white mixture by level tablespoonfuls, 2 inches apart, onto prepared baking sheets. Bake at 225° for 1 hour and 10 minutes. Turn oven off. Cool in oven 2 hours with oven door closed. Carefully remove cookies from paper; let cool on wire racks. Store in an airtight container. Yield: 4 dozen.

PER COOKIE: 12 CALORIES (8% FROM FAT)
FAT 0.1G (SATURATED FAT 0.0G)
PROTEIN 0.3G CARBOHYDRATE 2.7G
CHOLESTEROL 0MG SODIUM 5MG

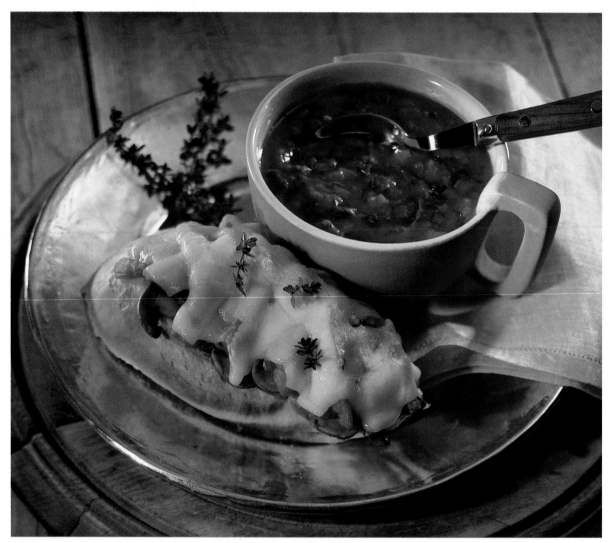

Mushroom and Roasted Pepper Sandwich and Spinach-Salsa Soup

VEGETARIAN LUNCH

Servings		*Calories*
1 serving	Mushroom and Roasted Pepper Sandwiches	225
1 cup	Spinach-Salsa Soup	165
1 cup	Sparkling mineral water	0

Serves 4
TOTAL CALORIES PER SERVING: 390
(CALORIES FROM FAT: 21%)

MUSHROOM AND ROASTED PEPPER SANDWICHES

Vegetable cooking spray
6 cups sliced fresh mushrooms
1½ teaspoons Worcestershire sauce
4 (1-inch-thick) diagonally cut Italian bread
     slices, lightly toasted (about 6 ounces)
½ cup drained water-packed roasted red bell
     peppers, cut into thin strips
4 (1-ounce) slices part-skim mozzarella cheese
Fresh thyme sprigs (optional)

Coat a large nonstick skillet with cooking spray, and place over medium-high heat until hot. Add mushrooms, and sauté 4 minutes or until lightly browned. Remove from heat, and stir in Worcestershire sauce.

Spoon about ⅓ cup mushroom mixture onto each bread slice; top each with one-fourth of pepper strips and 1 slice cheese.

Place sandwiches on a baking sheet, and broil 5½ inches from heat (with electric oven door partially opened) for 2 minutes or until cheese melts. Garnish with thyme, if desired. Yield: 4 servings.

PER SERVING: 225 CALORIES (22% FROM FAT)
FAT 5.6G (SATURATED FAT 3.0G)
PROTEIN 13.2G CARBOHYDRATE 31.3G
CHOLESTEROL 17MG SODIUM 478MG

SPINACH-SALSA SOUP

It's easier to cut the package of spinach in half while it's still partially frozen.

Vegetable cooking spray
1½ teaspoons olive oil
¾ cup chopped onion
1 clove garlic, minced
1½ cups commercial salsa
1 cup tomato juice
1 teaspoon sugar
2 (14.5-ounce) cans no-salt-added whole
     tomatoes, undrained and chopped
1 (10¾-ounce) can condensed reduced-fat,
     reduced-sodium tomato soup, undiluted
½ (10-ounce) package frozen chopped spinach

Coat a large Dutch oven with cooking spray; add olive oil, and place over medium-high heat until hot. Add onion and garlic; sauté 2 minutes. Add remaining ingredients; bring to a boil. Cover, reduce heat, and simmer 10 minutes or until thoroughly heated. Yield: 4 (1-cup) servings.

PER SERVING: 165 CALORIES (19% FROM FAT)
FAT 3.5G (SATURATED FAT 0.6G)
PROTEIN 5.7G CARBOHYDRATE 32.4G
CHOLESTEROL 0MG SODIUM 787MG

Low-Cal Desserts: Quick and Easy!

• Spoon fruit sherbet over a wedge of sweet ripe cantaloupe.

• Top lemon sorbet with fresh raspberries and pineapple chunks.

• Toss fresh strawberries with a mixture of orange juice concentrate, honey, and chopped mint.

• Drizzle honey, lime juice, and grated lemon rind over peaches, cantaloupe, or honeydew melon.

• Sprinkle freshly squeezed lime juice over cantaloupe, and then add chopped fresh mint.

• Top vanilla nonfat ice cream with no-sugar-added apricot conserve and gingersnap crumbs.

• Pour diet cream soda into a frosty mug, and top it with vanilla nonfat ice cream.

• Stir instant coffee granules into softened vanilla or chocolate nonfat ice cream.

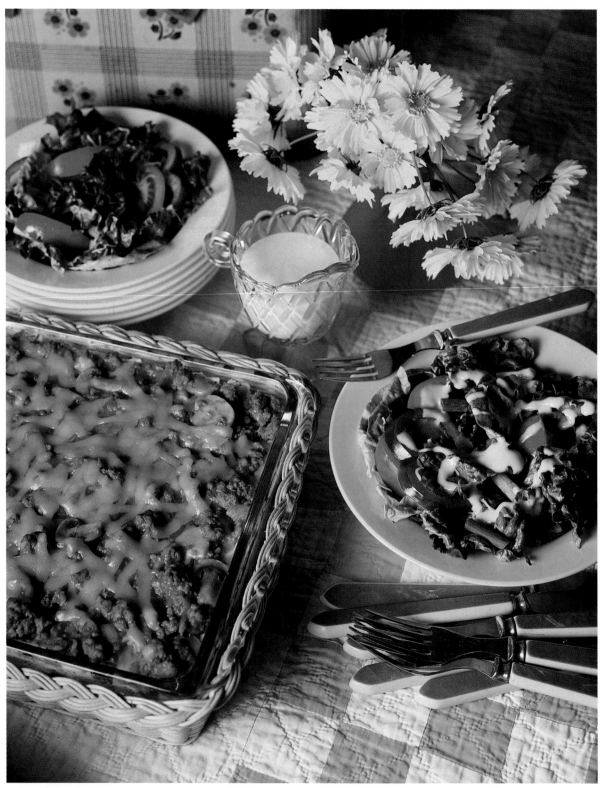

Ground Beef and Noodle Bake and Mixed Green Salad with Dijon Dressing (menu on page 66)

CASUAL SUPPERS

When the family gathers at the end of a busy day, you want to serve a meal everyone will enjoy. But that can be tricky if someone in the group is trying to lose weight.

To please them all, try meals featuring Ground Beef and Noodle Bake (page 66), Deep-Dish Pizza (page 69), or Mama's Chicken Stew (page 79). These are low in calories but big on taste.

Many of the menus suggest a dessert. The Hot Fudge Sundae (page 67) with only 193 calories can be enjoyed with any meal. Even the old-fashioned Peach Cobbler (page 76) can be yours without guilt. The secret is to cook the low-fat way and control your serving sizes.

FESTIVE FAMILY SUPPER

(pictured on page 64)

Servings		*Calories*
1 serving	Ground Beef and Noodle Bake	288
1 serving	Mixed Green Salad with Dijon Dressing	60
1 slice	Sesame-Onion Toast	110
1 serving	Hot Fudge Sundae	193

Serves 8
TOTAL CALORIES PER SERVING: 651
(CALORIES FROM FAT: 23%)

GROUND BEEF AND NOODLE BAKE

6 ounces medium egg noodles, uncooked
1 pound ground round
1 cup sliced fresh mushrooms
⅓ cup chopped onion
2 cloves garlic, minced
2 (8-ounce) cans no-salt-added tomato sauce
½ teaspoon freshly ground pepper
¼ teaspoon salt
1 (12-ounce) carton 1% low-fat cottage cheese
1 (8-ounce) carton nonfat sour cream
⅓ cup chopped green onions
2 tablespoons grated Parmesan cheese
1 tablespoon poppy seeds
¾ cup (3 ounces) shredded reduced-fat sharp
   Cheddar cheese, divided
Vegetable cooking spray

Cook noodles according to package directions, omitting salt and fat. Drain and set aside.

Cook meat, mushrooms, chopped onion, and minced garlic in a large nonstick skillet over medium heat until meat is browned, stirring until it crumbles. Drain and pat dry with paper towels. Wipe drippings from skillet with a paper towel. Return meat mixture to skillet. Add tomato sauce, pepper, and salt.

Combine cottage cheese, sour cream, green onions, Parmesan cheese, and poppy seeds in a large bowl. Stir in meat mixture, cooked noodles, and ¼ cup plus 2 tablespoons Cheddar cheese.

Coat a 2-quart baking dish with cooking spray. Place noodle mixture in dish. Cover and bake at 350° for 20 minutes. Uncover; sprinkle with remaining ¼ cup plus 2 tablespoons Cheddar cheese. Bake, uncovered, an additional 5 minutes. Yield: 8 servings.

PER SERVING: 288 CALORIES (24% FROM FAT)
FAT 7.8G (SATURATED FAT 3.2G)
PROTEIN 27.2G   CARBOHYDRATE 25.8G
CHOLESTEROL 65MG   SODIUM 400MG

MIXED GREEN SALAD WITH DIJON DRESSING

4 cups torn red leaf lettuce
4 cups torn Bibb lettuce
2 large tomatoes, cut into wedges
1 large green pepper, seeded and cut into rings
6 green onions, cut into 1-inch pieces
½ cup (2 ounces) finely shredded nonfat
   mozzarella cheese
Dijon Dressing

Combine first 6 ingredients in a large bowl, and toss gently. Serve salad with Dijon Dressing. Yield: 8 (1-cup) servings.

DIJON DRESSING

¼ cup nonfat mayonnaise
2 tablespoons water
1 tablespoon Dijon mustard
1 tablespoon honey
1 tablespoon cider vinegar
1½ teaspoons vegetable oil
⅛ teaspoon ground red pepper
1 clove garlic, crushed

Combine all ingredients in a small bowl. Whisk mixture vigorously until blended. Yield: ½ cup plus 2 tablespoons.

PER SERVING: 60 CALORIES (21% FROM FAT)
FAT 1.4G (SATURATED FAT 0.2G)
PROTEIN 3.5G   CARBOHYDRATE 9.7G
CHOLESTEROL 1MG   SODIUM 211MG

SESAME-ONION TOAST

2 tablespoons plus 2 teaspoons reduced-calorie margarine
2 teaspoons cider vinegar
8 (1-ounce) slices French bread
2 teaspoons sesame seeds
2 teaspoons instant minced onion
½ teaspoon garlic powder
½ teaspoon ground ginger
¼ teaspoon sugar
¼ teaspoon dried crushed red pepper

Combine margarine and vinegar in a small saucepan; cook over low heat until margarine is melted. Place bread slices on a baking sheet. Brush top side of each bread slice lightly with margarine mixture. Combine sesame seeds and remaining ingredients; sprinkle evenly over bread slices. Bake at 350° for 5 to 10 minutes or until bread slices are lightly browned. Yield: 8 slices.

PER SLICE: 110 CALORIES (28% FROM FAT)
FAT 3.4G (SATURATED FAT 0.6G)
PROTEIN 2.8G   CARBOHYDRATE 16.7G
CHOLESTEROL 1MG   SODIUM 202MG

HOT FUDGE SUNDAE

½ cup sugar
¼ cup unsweetened cocoa
1 tablespoon cornstarch
2 teaspoons instant coffee granules
½ cup plus 2 tablespoons evaporated skimmed milk
2 teaspoons margarine
½ teaspoon vanilla extract
4 cups low-fat vanilla ice cream
2 small bananas, sliced
2 teaspoons chopped pecans

Combine first 4 ingredients in a medium saucepan. Gradually stir in milk. Bring to a boil over medium heat, stirring constantly. Cook, stirring constantly, 1 minute or until thickened. Remove from heat.

Add margarine and vanilla, stirring until margarine melts.

To serve, scoop ½ cup low-fat vanilla ice cream into each individual bowl. Top ice cream evenly with hot fudge sauce, banana slices, and pecans. Yield: 8 servings.

PER SERVING: 193 CALORIES (20% FROM FAT)
FAT 4.3G (SATURATED FAT 2.0G)
PROTEIN 5.0G   CARBOHYDRATE 34.8G
CHOLESTEROL 10MG   SODIUM 90MG

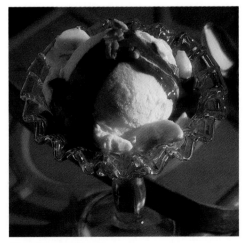

Hot Fudge Sundae

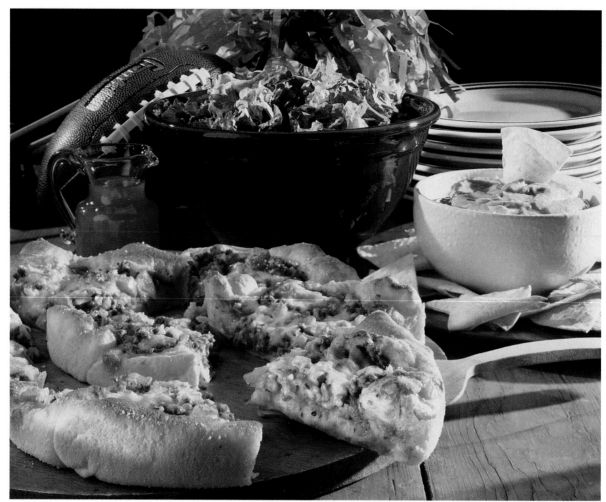

Deep-Dish Pizza, Salad with Vinaigrette Dressing, and Guacamole with Tortilla Chips

BEFORE THE GAME

Servings		*Calories*
1 serving	Guacamole with Tortilla Chips	90
1 serving	Deep-Dish Pizza	315
1 serving	Salad with Vinaigrette Dressing	17

Serves 8

TOTAL CALORIES PER SERVING: 422
(CALORIES FROM FAT: 25%)

GUACAMOLE WITH TORTILLA CHIPS

4 (6-inch) flour tortillas, each cut into 8 wedges
¾ cup peeled, cubed avocado
½ cup nonfat ricotta cheese
3 tablespoons coarsely chopped onion
1 tablespoon coarsely chopped fresh cilantro
1 tablespoon fresh lime juice
1½ teaspoons chopped jalapeño pepper
¼ teaspoon salt

Place tortilla wedges on a baking sheet; bake at 350° for 10 minutes or until crisp. Set aside.

Position knife blade in food processor bowl; add avocado and next 6 ingredients. Process until smooth. Spoon into a bowl; cover and chill. To serve, arrange 4 tortilla wedges around 2 tablespoons dip. Yield: 8 appetizer servings.

PER SERVING: 90 CALORIES (33% FROM FAT)
FAT 3.3G (SATURATED FAT 0.6G)
PROTEIN 3.6G   CARBOHYDRATE 13.7G
CHOLESTEROL 2MG   SODIUM 83MG

DEEP-DISH PIZZA

¾ cup water
½ cup no-salt-added tomato paste
1 teaspoon dried basil
½ teaspoon dried oregano
½ teaspoon fennel seeds, crushed
⅛ teaspoon ground red pepper
⅛ teaspoon black pepper
Vegetable cooking spray
6 ounces ground chuck
1 cup chopped onion
1 cup chopped green pepper
6 large cloves garlic, crushed
1 tablespoon cornmeal
2 (11-ounce) packages refrigerated French bread dough
¾ cup (3 ounces) shredded part-skim mozzarella cheese
¼ cup grated Romano cheese
Dried crushed red pepper (optional)

Combine first 7 ingredients in a small saucepan, stirring well; cook over low heat until thoroughly heated. Set aside.

Coat a large skillet with cooking spray, and place over medium-high heat until hot. Add meat and next 3 ingredients; cook until meat is browned, stirring until meat crumbles. Drain and set aside.

Coat 2 (9-inch) round cakepans with cooking spray, and sprinkle each with 1½ teaspoons cornmeal. Unroll 1 package bread dough; fold each corner in toward center to form a diamond shape. Pat dough, folded corners up, into a prepared pan. Repeat with remaining bread dough.

Spread ½ cup tomato mixture over each prepared crust; top each with 1 cup meat mixture. Sprinkle each with ¼ cup plus 2 tablespoons mozzarella cheese and 2 tablespoons Romano cheese. Bake at 475° for 12 minutes. Let stand 5 minutes. Cut each pizza into 4 wedges. Serve with crushed red pepper, if desired. Yield: 8 servings.

PER SERVING: 315 CALORIES (24% FROM FAT)
FAT 8.3G (SATURATED FAT 3.3G)
PROTEIN 15.3G   CARBOHYDRATE 43.8G
CHOLESTEROL 22MG   SODIUM 499MG

SALAD WITH VINAIGRETTE DRESSING

⅔ cup water
⅓ cup red wine vinegar
1 tablespoon sugar
1 teaspoon cornstarch
½ teaspoon fennel seeds, crushed
⅛ teaspoon garlic powder
8 cups tightly packed mixed salad greens

Combine water and next 5 ingredients in a non-aluminum saucepan; bring mixture to a boil over medium-high heat. Cook 1 minute or until thickened, stirring constantly. Serve warm or at room temperature over mixed salad greens. Yield: 8 servings.

PER SERVING: 17 CALORIES (5% FROM FAT)
FAT 0.1G (SATURATED FAT 0.0G)
PROTEIN 0.7G   CARBOHYDRATE 3.5G
CHOLESTEROL 0MG   SODIUM 4MG

FRIDAY NIGHT SPECIAL

Servings		*Calories*
1 serving	Garlicky Beef Fajitas	420
1 serving	Endive and Grape Salad	71
½ cup	Raspberry frozen yogurt	101

Serves 2

TOTAL CALORIES PER SERVING: 592
(CALORIES FROM FAT: 28%)

GARLICKY BEEF FAJITAS

6 ounces lean flank steak
1 teaspoon olive oil
1 small onion, halved lengthwise and thinly
    sliced (about ½ cup)
2 cups sliced fresh mushrooms
½ cup sweet red pepper strips
3 cloves garlic, minced
½ teaspoon ground cumin
⅛ teaspoon dried crushed red pepper
1 (8¾-ounce) can whole kernel corn, drained
1½ tablespoons fresh lime juice
2 (8-inch) flour tortillas
2 tablespoons nonfat sour cream

Trim fat from steak. Slice steak diagonally across grain into thin strips, and set aside.

Heat oil in a large nonstick skillet over medium-high heat. Add onion and next 3 ingredients; sauté 4 minutes or until tender. Remove vegetables from skillet; set aside.

Add steak to skillet; sauté 3 minutes or until done. Return vegetables to skillet. Add cumin, crushed red pepper, and corn; sauté 2 minutes or until thoroughly heated. Remove from heat; stir in lime juice. Divide mixture evenly between the tortillas; top each with 1 tablespoon sour cream. Yield: 2 servings.

PER SERVING: 420 CALORIES (30% FROM FAT)
FAT 13.8G (SATURATED FAT 4.3G)
PROTEIN 26.0G CARBOHYDRATE 51.4G
CHOLESTEROL 43MG SODIUM 541MG

ENDIVE AND GRAPE SALAD

1 tablespoon red wine vinegar
2 teaspoons water
1 teaspoon honey
½ teaspoon olive oil
¼ teaspoon Dijon mustard
⅛ teaspoon salt
⅛ teaspoon pepper
2 cups loosely packed torn curly endive
½ cup seedless red grapes, halved
1 tablespoon plus 1 teaspoon crumbled blue
    cheese

Combine first 7 ingredients in a small bowl; stir well with a wire whisk. Combine endive and grapes in a medium bowl. Add vinegar mixture; toss to coat. Sprinkle with blue cheese. Yield: 2 servings.

PER SERVING: 71 CALORIES (43% FROM FAT)
FAT 3.4G (SATURATED FAT 1.5G)
PROTEIN 2.3G CARBOHYDRATE 9.1G
CHOLESTEROL 5MG SODIUM 270MG

Menu Helper

While this menu suggests commercial frozen yogurt, it's easy and fun to make your own! Turn to page 134 for a basic vanilla, rich-tasting raspberry, and other fresh fruit varieties.

A NEIGHBORLY SUPPER

Servings		*Calories*
1 serving	Veal Parmigiana	310
1 cup	Cooked spaghetti	197
1 cup	Green salad	22
1 slice	French bread	82

Serves 6

TOTAL CALORIES PER SERVING: 611
(CALORIES FROM FAT: 17%)

VEAL PARMIGIANA

Vegetable cooking spray
½ cup chopped onion
2 teaspoons minced garlic
2 cups peeled, chopped tomato
2 (8-ounce) cans no-salt-added tomato sauce
¼ cup dry red wine
½ teaspoon dried oregano
1½ pounds veal cutlets
1 cup fine, dry breadcrumbs
2 tablespoons grated Parmesan cheese
¼ cup frozen egg substitute, thawed
1 tablespoon olive oil, divided
¾ cup (3 ounces) shredded part-skim
    mozzarella cheese

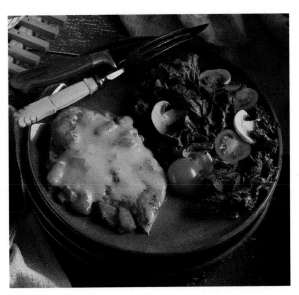

Veal Parmigiana

Coat a Dutch oven with cooking spray; place over medium-high heat until hot. Add onion and garlic; sauté until tender. Add tomato; cook 5 minutes, stirring frequently. Stir in tomato sauce, wine, and oregano. Cover and simmer 15 minutes. Remove from heat, and set aside.

Trim fat from cutlets. Place cutlets between 2 sheets of heavy-duty plastic wrap, and flatten to ¼-inch thickness, using a meat mallet or rolling pin. Combine breadcrumbs and Parmesan cheese in a shallow dish. Dip cutlets in egg substitute, and dredge in breadcrumb mixture. Place cutlets on wax paper; let stand 15 minutes.

Coat a large nonstick skillet with cooking spray; add 1½ teaspoons olive oil. Place over medium-high heat until hot. Add half of cutlets, and cook 4 to 5 minutes on each side or until lightly browned. Remove cutlets from skillet. Repeat procedure with remaining oil and cutlets.

Spoon ¾ cup tomato sauce mixture into a 13- x 9- x 2-inch baking dish coated with cooking spray. Place cutlets in dish, and top evenly with remaining sauce. Cover and bake at 350° for 25 minutes or until thoroughly heated. Sprinkle with mozzarella cheese. Bake, uncovered, an additional 8 minutes or until cheese melts. Yield: 6 servings.

PER SERVING: 310 CALORIES (28% FROM FAT)
FAT 9.5G (SATURATED FAT 3.2G)
PROTEIN 31.7G   CARBOHYDRATE 23.5G
CHOLESTEROL 104MG   SODIUM 356MG

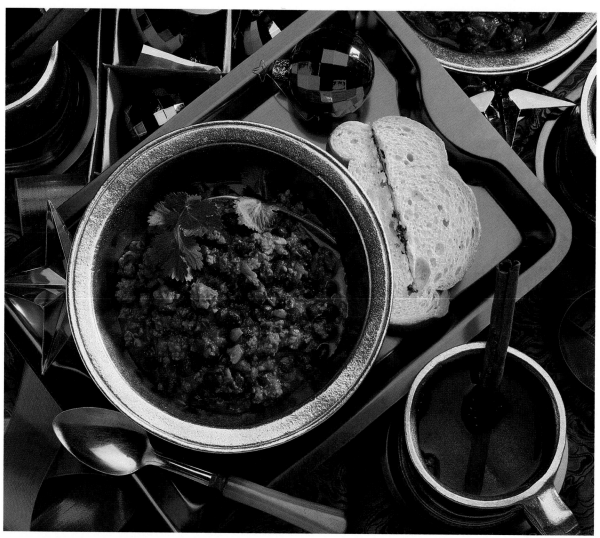

Lamb Chili with Black Beans and Two-Alarm Pepper Bread

COZY FIRESIDE DINING

Servings		*Calories*
1 serving	Lamb Chili with Black Beans	314
1 serving	Poppy Seed Coleslaw	36
1 serving	Two-Alarm Pepper Bread	98
¾ cup	Hot apple cider	87

Serves 8

TOTAL CALORIES PER SERVING: 535
(CALORIES FROM FAT: 18%)

LAMB CHILI WITH BLACK BEANS

1½ pounds lean ground lamb
1 cup chopped onion
2 cloves garlic, minced
2 (14½-ounce) cans no-salt-added whole
    tomatoes, undrained and chopped
1 cup dry red wine
1 tablespoon chili powder
1½ teaspoons ground cumin
1½ teaspoons dried oregano
1 teaspoon sugar
¼ teaspoon salt
3 (15-ounce) cans black beans, drained
¼ teaspoon hot sauce
Fresh cilantro sprigs (optional)

Combine first 3 ingredients in a Dutch oven; cook over medium heat until browned, stirring until meat crumbles. Drain in a colander; pat dry with paper towels. Wipe drippings from pan with a paper towel; return mixture to pan.

Add tomatoes and next 6 ingredients; bring to a boil. Cover, reduce heat, and simmer 2 hours, stirring occasionally. Stir in beans and hot sauce. Cover and simmer 30 minutes. Spoon into bowls; garnish with cilantro, if desired. Yield: 8 (1-cup) servings.

PER SERVING: 314 CALORIES (21% FROM FAT)
FAT 7.3G (SATURATED FAT 2.4G)
PROTEIN 29.9G CARBOHYDRATE 33.6G
CHOLESTEROL 61MG SODIUM 443MG

POPPY SEED COLESLAW

2 cups coarsely shredded red cabbage
2 cups coarsely shredded green cabbage
½ cup diagonally sliced celery
¼ cup minced purple onion
¼ cup white wine vinegar
2 tablespoons honey
1 teaspoon dry mustard
1 teaspoon vegetable oil
½ teaspoon salt
½ teaspoon poppy seeds

Combine first 4 ingredients in a large bowl. Combine vinegar and next 5 ingredients in a jar; cover tightly, and shake vigorously. Add to cabbage mixture, tossing gently to coat. Cover cabbage mixture, and chill up to 3 hours, stirring occasionally. Yield: 8 (½-cup) servings.

PER SERVING: 36 CALORIES (20% FROM FAT)
FAT 0.8G (SATURATED FAT 0.1G)
PROTEIN 0.6G CARBOHYDRATE 7.0G
CHOLESTEROL 0MG SODIUM 160MG

TWO-ALARM PEPPER BREAD

½ (16-ounce) loaf French bread
2 tablespoons reduced-calorie margarine,
    melted
2 teaspoons minced fresh parsley
¼ teaspoon dried crushed red pepper
⅛ teaspoon black pepper

Slice bread in half lengthwise. Combine margarine and next 3 ingredients. Spread over cut sides of bread; place cut sides together, and wrap in aluminum foil.

Bake at 350° for about 15 minutes or until thoroughly heated. Cut bread into 1-inch slices; serve warm. Yield: 8 servings.

PER SERVING: 98 CALORIES (22% FROM FAT)
FAT 2.4G (SATURATED FAT 0.4G)
PROTEIN 2.6G CARBOHYDRATE 15.8G
CHOLESTEROL 1MG SODIUM 192MG

Fat Burner

Stick to a 30-minute run or swim three times a week for a year, and you'll lose 12 pounds. That's without changing your eating habits. If you choose walking or aerobics, you'll lose 9 pounds. Spend the same amount of time weight-lifting, and you'll burn 5 pounds.

SUNDAY NIGHT SUPPER

Servings		Calories
1 serving	Pasta with Canadian Bacon	257
1 serving	Spinach Salad with Creamy Italian Dressing	50
2 sticks	Commercial breadsticks	82
1 serving	Peach Cobbler	228

Serves 4

TOTAL CALORIES PER SERVING: 617
(CALORIES FROM FAT: 18%)

PASTA WITH CANADIAN BACON

6 ounces penne (short tubular pasta), uncooked
Vegetable cooking spray
4 ounces Canadian bacon, chopped
¾ cup chopped sweet red pepper
¼ cup chopped onion
1 clove garlic, minced
1 (14½-ounce) can no-salt-added whole tomatoes, undrained and chopped
1 teaspoon sugar
½ teaspoon dried basil
¼ teaspoon freshly ground pepper
¼ teaspoon salt
2 teaspoons all-purpose flour
¼ cup evaporated skimmed milk
Fresh basil sprig (optional)

Cook pasta according to package directions, omitting salt and fat; drain and set aside.

Coat a large nonstick skillet with cooking spray; place over medium-high heat until hot. Add Canadian bacon and next 3 ingredients, and sauté until vegetables are tender. Add tomatoes and next 4 ingredients. Bring mixture to a boil. Cover, reduce heat, and simmer 10 minutes.

Combine flour and milk; stir well. Add flour mixture to tomato mixture, and cook over medium heat, stirring constantly, until slightly thickened.

Add pasta, stirring well. Cook over medium heat 2 to 3 minutes or until thoroughly heated. Transfer mixture to a serving bowl. Garnish with a basil sprig, if desired. Yield: 4 (1¼-cup) servings.

PER SERVING: 257 CALORIES (11% FROM FAT)
FAT 3.1G (SATURATED FAT 0.8G)
PROTEIN 13.9G   CARBOHYDRATE 43.4G
CHOLESTEROL 15MG   SODIUM 582MG

Focus on Fitness

For you to be truly fit, a program of aerobic exercise and weight training is necessary. Which is more important? Neither. Although weight, or strength, training can enhance just about every muscle group, it doesn't help the heart. And although an aerobic workout strengthens the heart, it doesn't provide important muscular and bone-building benefits.

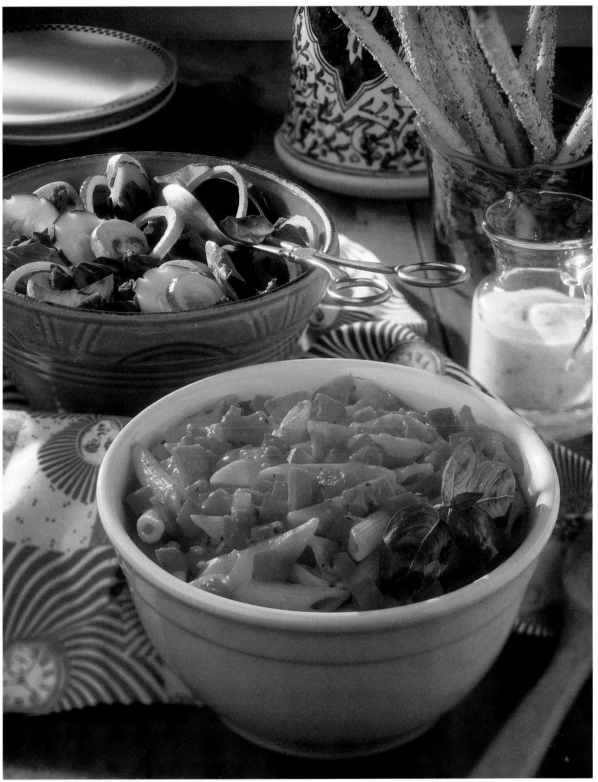

Pasta with Canadian Bacon and Spinach Salad with Creamy Italian Dressing

SPINACH SALAD WITH CREAMY ITALIAN DRESSING

½ cup (1 ounce) sun-dried tomatoes
1 cup hot water
½ medium cucumber
3 cups torn fresh spinach
½ small purple onion, sliced and separated
    into rings
½ cup sliced fresh mushrooms
Creamy Italian Dressing

Combine tomato and water in a small bowl; cover and let stand 15 minutes. Drain; coarsely chop tomato, and set aside.

Holding cucumber in one hand, run a citrus stripper or vegetable peeler lengthwise down the sides of cucumber to create strips about every ½ inch, if desired. Thinly slice cucumber.

Combine cucumber, tomato, spinach, onion, and mushrooms; toss gently. Arrange salad evenly on individual salad plates. Drizzle Creamy Italian Dressing evenly over each salad. Yield: 4 (1-cup) servings.

CREAMY ITALIAN DRESSING
3 tablespoons nonfat mayonnaise
2 tablespoons skim milk
1 tablespoon white wine vinegar
1 teaspoon grated Parmesan cheese
½ teaspoon sugar
¼ teaspoon dried basil
⅛ teaspoon dried Italian seasoning
1 clove garlic, crushed

Combine all ingredients in a small bowl; stir well with a wire whisk. Yield: ¼ cup plus 2 tablespoons.

PER SERVING: 50 CALORIES (9% FROM FAT)
FAT 0.5G (SATURATED FAT 0.2G)
PROTEIN 2.6G   CARBOHYDRATE 10.3G
CHOLESTEROL 0MG   SODIUM 322MG

PEACH COBBLER

3 cups peeled, sliced ripe fresh peaches (about
    1 pound)
Vegetable cooking spray
3 tablespoons sugar, divided
⅛ teaspoon ground cinnamon
1 cup all-purpose flour
1 teaspoon baking powder
¼ teaspoon salt
2 tablespoons stick margarine, cut into small
    pieces and chilled
¼ cup plus 1 tablespoon skim milk
¼ cup peach nectar
1 tablespoon margarine, melted

Arrange peaches in a 1-quart baking dish coated with cooking spray. Sprinkle with 2 tablespoons sugar and cinnamon; set aside. Combine flour, remaining 1 tablespoon sugar, baking powder, and salt in a bowl; cut in margarine with a pastry blender until mixture resembles coarse meal. Add milk, stirring until dry ingredients are moistened. Turn dough onto a lightly floured surface; knead lightly 2 to 3 times.

Roll dough to a ¼-inch thickness; cut with a 2½-inch biscuit cutter. Arrange pastry on top of peach mixture. Bake at 425° for 20 minutes.

Combine nectar and 1 tablespoon melted margarine in a saucepan; bring to boil. Pour over cobbler. Bake an additional 10 minutes. Serve warm. Yield: 4 (¾-cup) servings.

PER SERVING: 228 CALORIES (27% FROM FAT)
FAT 6.8G (SATURATED FAT 1.3G)
PROTEIN 3.4G   CARBOHYDRATE 40.0G
CHOLESTEROL 0MG   SODIUM 214MG

HARVEST PORK SUPPER

Servings		_Calories_
1 serving	Maple-Glazed Pork with Apples	352
1 medium	Seasoned baked sweet potatoes	165
1 cup	Steamed green beans	34

Serves 4

TOTAL CALORIES PER SERVING: 551
(CALORIES FROM FAT: 27%)

MAPLE-GLAZED PORK WITH APPLES

⅓ cup maple syrup
1 tablespoon spicy brown mustard
¼ teaspoon salt
¼ teaspoon pepper
¼ cup fine, dry breadcrumbs
4 (4-ounce) pork cutlets
2 teaspoons olive oil
½ cup unsweetened apple cider
2 medium Golden Delicious apples, each cored
    and cut into 16 wedges
2 tablespoons chopped fresh parsley

Combine first 4 ingredients in a small bowl; stir well with a wire whisk, and set aside. Place bread-crumbs in a large zip-top plastic bag. Add pork; seal bag, and shake to coat pork with breadcrumbs.

Heat oil in a large nonstick skillet over medium heat. Add pork, and cook 2 minutes on each side or until golden brown. Add cider and apple wedges; bring to a boil. Reduce heat, and simmer, uncovered, 10 minutes or until pork is done. Add maple syrup mixture, and cook 5 minutes or until thick and syrupy. Sprinkle with parsley. Yield: 4 servings.

PER SERVING: 352 CALORIES (29% FROM FAT)
FAT 11.2G (SATURATED FAT 3.5G)
PROTEIN 26.2G   CARBOHYDRATE 36.4G
CHOLESTEROL 72MG   SODIUM 308MG

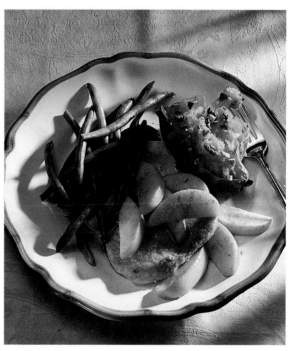

Maple-Glazed Pork with Apples

Menu Helper

The nutrient analysis for each medium-size sweet potato includes 2 teaspoons reduced-calorie margarine and 1 teaspoon toasted, chopped pecans.

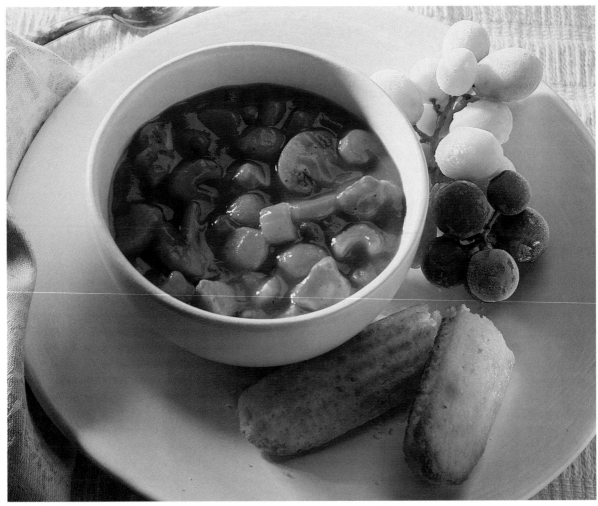

Mama's Chicken Stew and Buttermilk Corn Sticks

SLOW-COOKING STEW

Servings		*Calories*
1½ cups	Mama's Chicken Stew	257
1 stick	Buttermilk Corn Sticks	88
1 cup	Frosted grapes	114
1 cup	Cranberry-Raspberry Tea	95

Serves 8

TOTAL CALORIES PER SERVING: 554
(CALORIES FROM FAT: 12%)

MAMA'S CHICKEN STEW

1 pound skinned, boned chicken breasts, cut into bite-size pieces
1 pound skinned, boned chicken thighs, cut into bite-size pieces
2 cups water
2 cups halved mushrooms
1 cup frozen small whole onions
1 cup (½-inch) sliced celery
1 cup thinly sliced carrot
1 teaspoon paprika
½ teaspoon salt
½ teaspoon rubbed sage
½ teaspoon dried thyme
½ teaspoon pepper
1 (14¼-ounce) can fat-free chicken broth
1 (6-ounce) can tomato paste
¼ cup water
3 tablespoons cornstarch
2 cups frozen English peas

Combine first 14 ingredients in an electric slow cooker. Cover; cook on high-heat setting 4 hours or until carrot is tender. Combine ¼ cup water and cornstarch in a bowl. Add cornstarch mixture and peas to slow cooker; stir well. Cover; cook on high-heat 30 minutes. Yield: 8 (1½-cup) servings.

PER SERVING: 257 CALORIES (12% FROM FAT)
FAT 3.5G (SATURATED FAT 0.8G)
PROTEIN 30.8G CARBOHYDRATE 25.1G
CHOLESTEROL 78MG SODIUM 359MG

BUTTERMILK CORN STICKS

⅔ cup yellow cornmeal
½ cup all-purpose flour
¾ teaspoon baking powder
½ teaspoon baking soda
¼ teaspoon salt
¼ teaspoon paprika
¾ cup nonfat buttermilk
2 tablespoons sugar
2 tablespoons vegetable oil
1 egg, lightly beaten
Vegetable cooking spray

Combine first 6 ingredients in a medium bowl; make a well in center of mixture.
Combine buttermilk and next 3 ingredients; add to dry ingredients, stirring just until moistened.
Place cast-iron corn stick pans coated with cooking spray in a 425° oven for 3 minutes or until hot. Remove pans from oven; spoon batter into pans, filling two-thirds full. Bake at 425° for 10 minutes or until lightly browned. Yield: 1 dozen.

PER CORN STICK: 88 CALORIES (31% FROM FAT)
FAT 3.0G (SATURATED FAT 0.6G)
PROTEIN 2.3G CARBOHYDRATE 13.0G
CHOLESTEROL 19MG SODIUM 124MG

CRANBERRY-RASPBERRY TEA

This tea is delightful when served warm, but it's also a refreshing thirst-quencher when poured over ice.

5 cups water
12 regular-size tea bags
3 cups cranberry-raspberry-strawberry juice blend
¼ cup honey

Bring water to a boil in a saucepan. Add tea bags; remove from heat. Cover and steep 5 minutes. Remove and discard tea bags. Add juice blend and honey; stir well.
Serve warm or chilled. Yield: 8 (1-cup) servings.

PER SERVING: 95 CALORIES (0% FROM FAT)
FAT 0.0G (SATURATED FAT 0.0G)
PROTEIN 0.1G CARBOHYDRATE 24.9G
CHOLESTEROL 0MG SODIUM 7MG

Frosted Grapes

Wash seedless grapes, and freeze for 45 minutes; let stand at least 2 minutes before serving.

Down Memory Lane

Servings		Calories
1 serving	Simple Baked Chicken	235
1 serving	Stewed Tomatoes and Onions	37
1 serving	Basil Mashed Potatoes	136
2 tablespoons	Home-Style Gravy	10
½ cup	Fruit sherbet	132

Serves 6
Total Calories per Serving: 550
(Calories from Fat: 17%)

Simple Baked Chicken

This easy chicken dish gets its spark from lemonade concentrate and lots of freshly ground pepper.

1 (3-pound) broiler-fryer, cut up and skinned
Vegetable cooking spray
½ cup frozen lemonade concentrate, thawed
  and undiluted
2 tablespoons canned low-sodium chicken
  broth, undiluted
½ teaspoon garlic powder
1 teaspoon dried rosemary, crushed
1 teaspoon freshly ground pepper

Place chicken on a rack in a roasting pan coated with cooking spray.

Combine lemonade concentrate, chicken broth, and garlic powder, stirring well. Sprinkle chicken with rosemary and pepper; brush with some of lemonade mixture.

Bake at 400° for 45 to 50 minutes or until chicken is done, turning and basting occasionally with remaining lemonade mixture. Yield: 6 servings.

Per Serving: 235 Calories (29% from Fat)
Fat 7.5g (Saturated Fat 2.0g)
Protein 28.6g Carbohydrate 12.1g
Cholesterol 87mg Sodium 87mg

Stewed Tomatoes and Onions

Vegetable cooking spray
½ cup chopped green pepper
¼ cup thinly sliced celery
1 small onion, thinly sliced and separated into
  rings
1 clove garlic, minced
3 cups peeled, coarsely chopped tomato
1 tablespoon red wine vinegar
2 teaspoons sugar
⅛ teaspoon pepper

Coat a large nonstick skillet with cooking spray; place over medium-high heat until hot. Add green pepper, celery, onion, and garlic; sauté 5 minutes or until vegetables are tender. Add tomato and remaining ingredients; bring to a boil. Cover, reduce heat, and simmer 15 minutes, stirring occasionally. Yield: 6 (½-cup) servings.

Per Serving: 37 Calories (12% from Fat)
Fat 0.5g (Saturated Fat 0.1g)
Protein 1.2g Carbohydrate 8.3g
Cholesterol 0mg Sodium 14mg

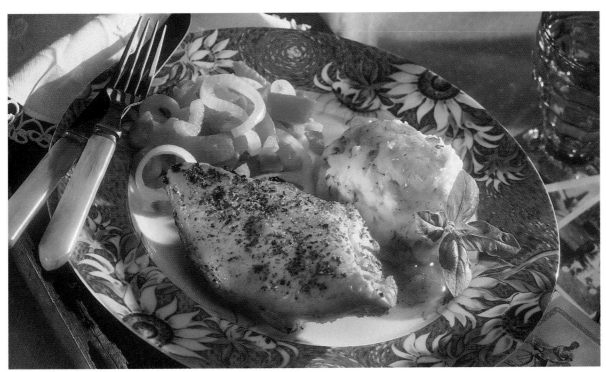

Simple Baked Chicken, Stewed Tomatoes and Onions, and Basil Mashed Potatoes with Home-Style Gravy

BASIL MASHED POTATOES

5 cups peeled, sliced baking potato
¼ cup plus 2 tablespoons skim milk
¼ cup plain nonfat yogurt
½ teaspoon salt
¼ teaspoon ground white pepper
3 tablespoons minced fresh basil
Fresh basil sprigs (optional)

Place potato in a large saucepan; add water to cover. Bring to a boil; cook 15 minutes or until tender. Drain potato, and place in a large bowl. Beat at medium speed of an electric mixer 1 minute or until smooth.

Combine milk and next 3 ingredients; gradually add milk mixture to potato, beating at medium speed until smooth. Stir in minced basil. Garnish with fresh basil sprigs, if desired. Yield: 6 (1-cup) servings.

PER SERVING: 136 CALORIES (1% FROM FAT)
FAT 0.2G (SATURATED FAT 0.0G)
PROTEIN 4.4G   CARBOHYDRATE 30.0G
CHOLESTEROL 0MG   SODIUM 220MG

HOME-STYLE GRAVY

Vegetable cooking spray
½ cup chopped onion
1 teaspoon dried thyme
1½ tablespoons cornstarch
¼ cup water
1¼ cups canned low-sodium chicken broth
¼ teaspoon salt
¼ teaspoon pepper
¼ teaspoon poultry seasoning

Coat a medium saucepan with cooking spray, and place over medium-high heat until hot. Add onion and thyme; sauté 3 minutes. Combine cornstarch and water, stirring until smooth; stir in broth. Add cornstarch mixture, salt, pepper, and poultry seasoning to onion mixture. Bring to a boil over medium heat, stirring constantly. Cook, stirring constantly, until thickened and bubbly. Yield: 1½ cups.

PER TABLESPOON: 5 CALORIES (18% FROM FAT)
FAT 0.1G (SATURATED FAT 0.0G)
PROTEIN 0.2G   CARBOHYDRATE 0.9G
CHOLESTEROL 0MG   SODIUM 29MG

SUNSET SUPPER

Servings		*Calories*
1 serving	Turkey Jalapeño	335
1 serving	Snow Pea Stir-Fry	69
1 serving	Seasoned Vermicelli and Rice	141

Serves 4

TOTAL CALORIES PER SERVING: 545
(CALORIES FROM FAT: 16%)

TURKEY JALAPEÑO

1 pound turkey breast cutlets
⅓ cup all-purpose flour
½ teaspoon freshly ground pepper
2 teaspoons vegetable oil
Vegetable cooking spray
¼ cup sliced green onions
½ teaspoon peeled, minced gingerroot
½ cup red jalapeño jelly
¼ cup unsweetened apple juice
1 tablespoon red wine vinegar
1 teaspoon low-sodium Worcestershire sauce
2 teaspoons cornstarch
1 tablespoon water
Green onion curls (optional)

Place cutlets between 2 sheets of heavy-duty plastic wrap, and flatten to ⅛-inch thickness, using a meat mallet or rolling pin. Combine flour and pepper; dredge turkey cutlets in flour mixture.

Heat oil in a large nonstick skillet over medium heat until hot. Add cutlets, and cook 3 to 4 minutes on each side or until done. Transfer to a platter, and keep warm. Wipe drippings from skillet.

Coat skillet with cooking spray, and place over medium-high heat until hot. Add sliced green onions and gingerroot; sauté until tender. Add jelly and next 3 ingredients. Reduce heat, and cook until jelly melts and mixture is thoroughly heated.

Combine cornstarch and water; stir until smooth. Add to jelly mixture. Cook, stirring constantly,

until thickened and bubbly. Spoon sauce over turkey cutlets; garnish with green onion curls, if desired. Yield: 4 servings.

PER SERVING: 335 CALORIES (16% FROM FAT)
FAT 5.9G (SATURATED FAT 1.5G)
PROTEIN 31.3G CARBOHYDRATE 38.3G
CHOLESTEROL 70MG SODIUM 84MG

SNOW PEA STIR-FRY

Vegetable cooking spray
1 teaspoon dark sesame oil
½ cup diagonally sliced carrot
2 (6-ounce) packages frozen snow pea pods
¼ cup sliced water chestnuts
½ cup canned low-sodium chicken broth,
   undiluted
2 teaspoons low-sodium soy sauce
1 teaspoon cornstarch

Coat a large nonstick skillet with cooking spray; add oil. Place over medium-high heat until hot. Add carrot; sauté 2 minutes.

Add snow peas, water chestnuts, and broth; bring to a boil. Cover, reduce heat, and simmer 2 to 3 minutes or until vegetables are crisp-tender.

Combine soy sauce and cornstarch; add to vegetable mixture. Cook over medium heat, stirring constantly, until thickened. Yield: 4 (½-cup) servings.

PER SERVING: 69 CALORIES (22% FROM FAT)
FAT 1.7G (SATURATED FAT 0.2G)
PROTEIN 3.4G CARBOHYDRATE 10.4G
CHOLESTEROL 0MG SODIUM 100MG

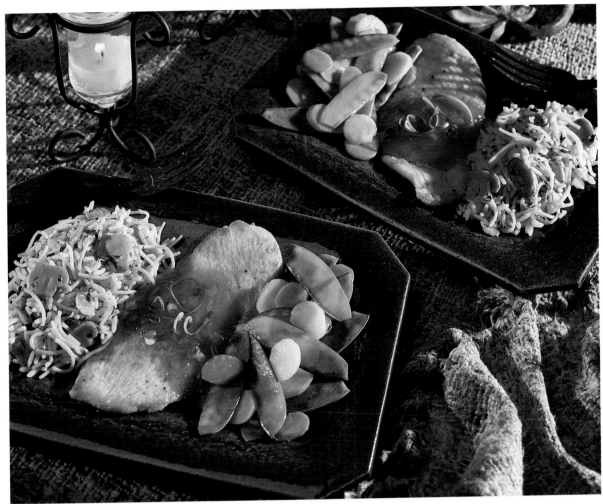

Turkey Jalapeño, Snow Pea Stir-Fry, and Seasoned Vermicelli and Rice

SEASONED VERMICELLI AND RICE

1½ teaspoons margarine
½ cup chopped onion
½ cup instant long-grain rice, uncooked
2 ounces vermicelli, uncooked and broken into
    1-inch pieces
1¼ cups water
1 (4-ounce) can sliced mushrooms, drained
1½ teaspoons chicken-flavored bouillon
    granules
½ teaspoon dried oregano
½ teaspoon dried thyme
⅛ teaspoon freshly ground pepper
2 tablespoons chopped fresh parsley

Melt margarine in a saucepan over medium-high heat. Add onion; sauté until tender. Add rice and vermicelli; sauté, stirring constantly, 3 to 5 minutes or until rice and pasta are lightly browned.

Add water and next 5 ingredients to rice mixture, stirring well. Bring to a boil; cover, reduce heat, and simmer 10 minutes or until rice and pasta are tender and liquid is absorbed. Fluff with a fork, and stir in parsley. Yield: 4 (½-cup) servings.

PER SERVING: 141 CALORIES (14% FROM FAT)
FAT 2.2G (SATURATED FAT 0.5G)
PROTEIN 3.5G CARBOHYDRATE 27.0G
CHOLESTEROL 0MG SODIUM 382MG

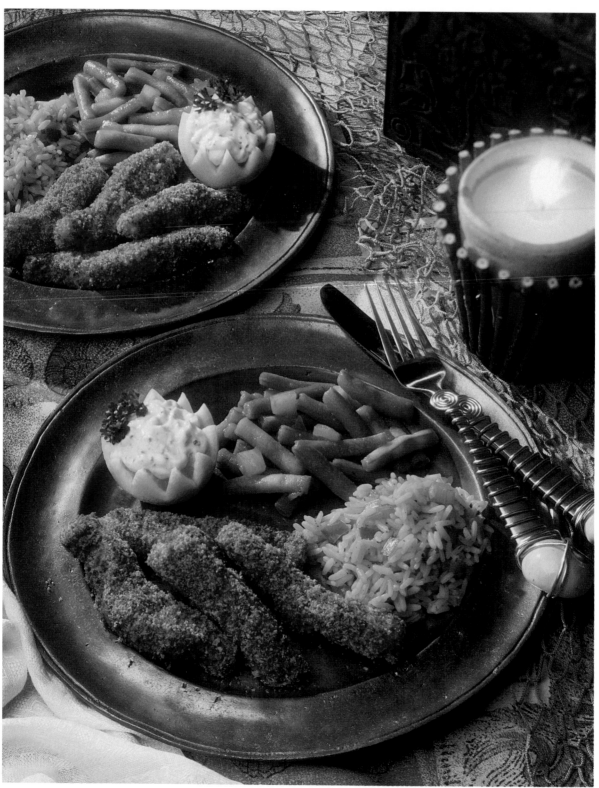

Grouper Fingers with Lemon-Pepper Mayonnaise, Green Beans in Tomato Sauce, and Savory Rice

A FAMILY AFFAIR

Servings		Calories
1 serving	Grouper Fingers with Lemon-Pepper Mayonnaise	147
1 serving	Green Beans in Tomato Sauce	59
1 serving	Savory Rice	148
½ cup	Tropical Frozen Yogurt	97

Serves 6
TOTAL CALORIES PER SERVING: 451
(CALORIES FROM FAT: 12%)

GROUPER FINGERS WITH LEMON-PEPPER MAYONNAISE

1½ pounds grouper fillets
¼ cup nonfat mayonnaise
1 tablespoon water
¾ teaspoon grated lemon rind
1 tablespoon lemon juice
¾ cup soft whole wheat breadcrumbs, toasted
1 teaspoon coarsely ground pepper
¾ teaspoon garlic powder
Vegetable cooking spray
3 lemons (optional)
Lemon-Pepper Mayonnaise
Fresh parsley sprigs (optional)

Cut fillets diagonally into 1-inch-wide strips. Combine ¼ cup mayonnaise and next 3 ingredients; stir well. Brush both sides of strips with mayonnaise mixture.

Combine breadcrumbs, pepper, and garlic powder. Dredge strips in breadcrumb mixture. Place on a baking sheet coated with cooking spray.

Bake at 425° for 25 minutes or until fish is golden and flakes easily when tested with a fork.

Using a small sharp knife, make continuous V-shaped cuts into the centers and around the middles of 3 lemons, if desired. Gently twist halves apart. Spoon 1 tablespoon of Lemon-Pepper Mayonnaise into each lemon crown, and top each with a parsley sprig, if desired. Yield: 6 servings.

LEMON-PEPPER MAYONNAISE

¼ cup plus 2 tablespoons nonfat mayonnaise
2 teaspoons skim milk
1 teaspoon grated lemon rind
1 teaspoon lemon juice
¾ teaspoon coarsely ground pepper
¼ teaspoon garlic powder

Combine all ingredients; stir well. Cover; chill thoroughly. Yield: ¼ cup plus 2 tablespoons.

PER SERVING: 147 CALORIES (9% FROM FAT)
FAT 1.5G (SATURATED FAT 0.3G)
PROTEIN 22.9G   CARBOHYDRATE 9.6G
CHOLESTEROL 42MG   SODIUM 416MG

FYI

Do you really need to drink eight glasses of water a day? Yes, and maybe even more if you are exercising. During workouts, keep a water bottle handy so you can drink before, during, and after exercise. The water will keep your body cool and hydrated.

GREEN BEANS IN TOMATO SAUCE

2 teaspoons olive oil
1 cup chopped onion
1 large clove garlic, minced
2 (10-ounce) packages frozen green beans
1 (8-ounce) can no-salt-added tomato sauce
¼ cup water
⅛ teaspoon salt
Dash of freshly ground pepper
Dash of ground cinnamon

Heat oil in a large nonstick skillet over medium-high heat until hot. Add onion and garlic, and sauté until onion is tender.

Add beans and next 3 ingredients. Bring to a boil; reduce heat, and simmer, uncovered, 8 to 10 minutes or until beans are tender, stirring occasionally. Add pepper and cinnamon; stir well. Yield: 6 (½-cup) servings.

PER SERVING: 59 CALORIES (26% FROM FAT)
FAT 1.7G (SATURATED FAT 0.3G)
PROTEIN 1.9G   CARBOHYDRATE 10.3G
CHOLESTEROL 0MG   SODIUM 67MG

SAVORY RICE

½ teaspoon salt
½ teaspoon paprika
½ teaspoon dried Italian seasoning
¼ teaspoon ground red pepper
¼ teaspoon freshly ground black pepper
Vegetable cooking spray
1 tablespoon reduced-calorie stick margarine
⅔ cup chopped onion
⅔ cup chopped celery
⅔ cup chopped green pepper
1 clove garlic, minced
1 cup long-grain rice, uncooked
2 cups canned no-salt-added chicken broth, undiluted

Combine first 5 ingredients in a small bowl; stir well, and set aside.

Coat a large saucepan with cooking spray; add margarine. Place over medium-high heat until margarine melts. Add onion and next 3 ingredients; sauté until vegetables are crisp-tender.

Stir in rice; sauté until rice is lightly browned. Stir in seasoning mixture and chicken broth. Bring to a boil; cover, reduce heat, and simmer 20 to 25 minutes or until rice is tender and liquid is absorbed. Yield: 6 (½-cup) servings.

PER SERVING: 148 CALORIES (14% FROM FAT)
FAT 2.3G (SATURATED FAT 0.4G)
PROTEIN 3.3G   CARBOHYDRATE 27.8G
CHOLESTEROL 0MG   SODIUM 273MG

TROPICAL FROZEN YOGURT

Spoon leftovers into freezer-safe containers, and store in freezer.

2 cups fresh strawberry halves
2 cups peeled, sliced banana
¼ cup sugar
¾ cup frozen pineapple juice concentrate, thawed and undiluted
½ cup plain low-fat yogurt

Position knife blade in food processor bowl; add first 4 ingredients. Process until smooth, scraping sides of processor bowl once. Add yogurt, and pulse 3 or 4 times or until combined.

Pour mixture into freezer can of a 2-quart hand-turned or electric freezer. Freeze according to manufacturer's instructions. Pack freezer with additional ice and rock salt, and let stand 1 hour before serving. Scoop frozen yogurt into individual dessert bowls, and serve immediately. Yield: 11 (½-cup) servings.

PER SERVING: 97 CALORIES (4% FROM FAT)
FAT 0.4G (SATURATED FAT 0.2G)
PROTEIN 1.3G   CARBOHYDRATE 23.3G
CHOLESTEROL 1MG   SODIUM 8MG

FROM THE PANTRY

Servings		*Calories*
1 serving	Oriental Tuna Patties	131
1 serving	Tangy Snow Peas and Peaches	49
1 slice	Pound cake	80
½ cup	Fruit cocktail	50

Serves 4
TOTAL CALORIES PER SERVING: 310
(CALORIES FROM FAT: 8%)

ORIENTAL TUNA PATTIES

Vegetable cooking spray
⅓ cup sliced green onions
⅓ cup chopped celery
2 cloves garlic, minced
1 (12½-ounce) can chunk white tuna in spring
    water, well drained
¼ cup fine, dry breadcrumbs
¼ cup frozen egg substitute, thawed
2 tablespoons low-sodium soy sauce
½ teaspoon grated gingerroot
¼ teaspoon prepared horseradish

Coat a large nonstick skillet with cooking spray; place over medium-high heat until hot. Add green onions, celery, and garlic; sauté until tender.

Combine sautéed vegetables, tuna, and remaining ingredients in a large bowl; stir well. Cover and chill 15 minutes. Shape mixture into 4 patties.

Coat skillet with cooking spray, and place over medium-high heat until hot. Add patties, and cook 3 minutes on each side or until lightly browned. Yield: 4 servings.

PER SERVING: 131 CALORIES (16% FROM FAT)
FAT 2.3G (SATURATED FAT 0.5G)
PROTEIN 19.1G   CARBOHYDRATE 6.7G
CHOLESTEROL 26MG   SODIUM 528MG

TANGY SNOW PEAS AND PEACHES

1 (8¾-ounce) can peach slices in juice,
    undrained
1 (10-ounce) package frozen snow pea pods
¾ teaspoon Dijon mustard
⅛ teaspoon pepper

Drain peaches, reserving 2 tablespoons juice.

Cook snow peas according to package directions, omitting salt and fat. Drain. Combine reserved 2 tablespoons juice, mustard, and pepper; pour over peas. Add reserved peaches; cook until thoroughly heated. Yield: 4 servings.

PER SERVING: 49 CALORIES (6% FROM FAT)
FAT 0.3G (SATURATED FAT 0.0G)
PROTEIN 2.6G   CARBOHYDRATE 9.7G
CHOLESTEROL 0MG   SODIUM 33MG

Quick Tip

For dessert, spoon chilled unsweetened fruit cocktail over nonfat pound cake. Or process undrained fruit cocktail in a food processor until smooth. Freeze the mixture in a shallow pan; then return it to the processor bowl to process until it's the consistency of sherbet.

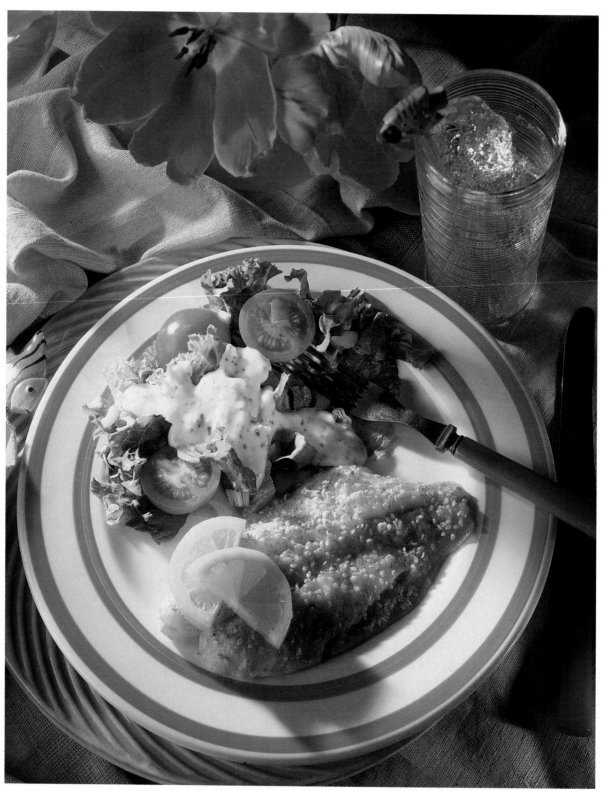

Baked Orange Roughy and Tossed Salad with Buttermilk Dressing

EASY FISH SUPPER

Servings		Calories
1 serving	Baked Orange Roughy	92
1 serving	Tossed Salad with Buttermilk Dressing	42
1 small	Baked potato	110
1 cup	Fresh blueberries	82

Serves 6
TOTAL CALORIES PER SERVING: 326
(CALORIES FROM FAT: 9%)

BAKED ORANGE ROUGHY

6 (4-ounce) orange roughy fillets
2 tablespoons water
1 teaspoon peeled, minced gingerroot
½ teaspoon lemon juice
½ teaspoon low-sodium soy sauce
¼ teaspoon dried crushed red pepper
1 clove garlic, minced
2 tablespoons sesame seeds, toasted
Vegetable cooking spray
¼ teaspoon paprika
Lemon slices (optional)

Place fillets in a shallow baking dish. Combine water and next 5 ingredients in container of an electric blender; cover and process until smooth. Pour over fillets. Cover and marinate in refrigerator 1 to 2 hours.

Remove fillets from marinade; discard marinade. Coat both sides of each fillet with sesame seeds. Place fillets on rack of a broiler pan coated with cooking spray.

Broil 3½ inches from heat (with electric oven door partially opened) 6 minutes or until fish flakes easily when tested with a fork. Sprinkle with paprika; garnish with lemon, if desired. Yield: 6 servings.

PER SERVING: 92 CALORIES (21% FROM FAT)
FAT 2.1G (SATURATED FAT 0.2G)
PROTEIN 16.6G CARBOHYDRATE 1.0G
CHOLESTEROL 22MG SODIUM 81MG

TOSSED SALAD WITH BUTTERMILK DRESSING

2 cups tightly packed torn romaine lettuce
2 cups tightly packed torn leaf lettuce
1¼ cups halved cherry tomatoes
½ cup sliced purple onion
¼ cup chopped celery
Buttermilk Dressing

Combine first 5 ingredients in a large bowl; toss well. Divide salad mixture among 6 plates, and top with Buttermilk Dressing. Yield: 6 servings.

BUTTERMILK DRESSING
½ cup nonfat buttermilk
¼ cup plus 2 tablespoons nonfat mayonnaise
1 tablespoon grated Parmesan cheese
1 teaspoon dried parsley flakes
¼ teaspoon cracked pepper
1 clove garlic, minced

Combine all ingredients in a small bowl; stir well. Yield: ¾ cup plus 2 tablespoons.

PER SERVING: 42 CALORIES (11% FROM FAT)
FAT 0.5G (SATURATED FAT 0.3G)
PROTEIN 2.1G CARBOHYDRATE 7.8G
CHOLESTEROL 1MG SODIUM 239MG

VEGETARIAN SUPPER FOR TWO

Servings		_Calories_
1 serving	Italian Salad Toss	62
1 serving	Mushroom Marinara	287
1 serving	Dilled Fresh Squash	36
1 slice	Italian bread	78

Serves 2
TOTAL CALORIES PER SERVING: 463
(CALORIES FROM FAT: 17%)

ITALIAN SALAD TOSS

1 cup torn romaine lettuce
¼ cup frozen artichoke hearts, thawed and
   quartered
2 tablespoons (½ ounce) shredded part-skim
   mozzarella cheese
2 thin slices purple onion, separated into rings
2 cherry tomatoes, quartered
1 small sweet banana pepper, seeded and
   coarsely chopped
2 tablespoons commercial reduced-calorie
   Italian dressing
2 teaspoons red wine vinegar
1½ teaspoons chopped walnuts, toasted

Combine first 6 ingredients in a medium bowl;
toss well.
Combine Italian dressing and red wine vinegar;
pour over lettuce mixture, tossing gently. Arrange
lettuce mixture evenly on individual serving plates,
and sprinkle each with ¾ teaspoon chopped walnuts. Yield: 2 servings.

PER SERVING: 62 CALORIES (41% FROM FAT)
FAT 2.8G (SATURATED FAT 0.9G)
PROTEIN 3.8G CARBOHYDRATE 6.5G
CHOLESTEROL 4MG SODIUM 263MG

MUSHROOM MARINARA

Vegetable cooking spray
1 teaspoon olive oil
2 cups sliced fresh mushrooms
1 (14¼-ounce) can no-salt-added stewed
   tomatoes, undrained and coarsely chopped
¼ cup no-salt-added tomato paste
1 tablespoon dried parsley flakes
1 tablespoon dry red wine
½ teaspoon dried oregano
½ teaspoon dried basil
¼ teaspoon dried thyme
¼ teaspoon pepper
⅛ teaspoon salt
⅛ teaspoon garlic powder
3 ounces angel hair pasta, uncooked
1 teaspoon grated Parmesan cheese

Coat a medium saucepan with cooking spray;
add olive oil. Place over medium-high heat until
hot. Add mushrooms, and sauté until tender.
Add stewed tomatoes and next 9 ingredients; stir
well. Bring to a boil; reduce heat and simmer,
uncovered, 5 to 10 minutes, stirring occasionally.
Cook pasta according to package directions,
omitting salt and fat. Drain. Top each serving with
mushroom mixture. Sprinkle each with ½ teaspoon
cheese. Yield: 2 servings.

PER SERVING: 287 CALORIES (12% FROM FAT)
FAT 3.9G (SATURATED FAT 0.6G)
PROTEIN 10.9G CARBOHYDRATE 55.0G
CHOLESTEROL 1MG SODIUM 220MG

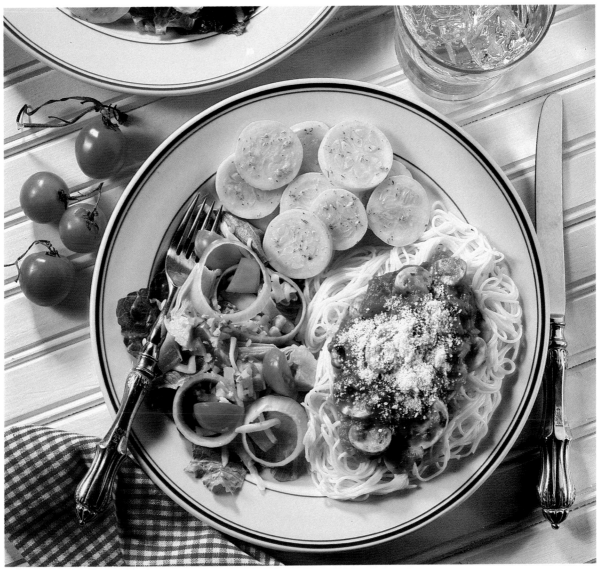

Mushroom Marinara, Italian Salad Toss, and Dilled Fresh Squash

DILLED FRESH SQUASH

1½ cups sliced yellow squash
2 teaspoons lemon juice
1 teaspoon margarine, melted
⅛ teaspoon salt
⅛ teaspoon dried dillweed
Dash of pepper

Arrange squash in a vegetable steamer over boiling water. Cover and steam 2 to 3 minutes or until squash is crisp-tender. Transfer squash to a serving bowl, and keep warm.

Combine lemon juice and next 4 ingredients; pour lemon juice mixture over squash, and toss gently. Yield: 2 servings.

PER SERVING: 36 CALORIES (53% FROM FAT)
FAT 2.1G (SATURATED FAT 0.4G)
PROTEIN 1.0G   CARBOHYDRATE 4.2G
CHOLESTEROL 0MG   SODIUM 171MG

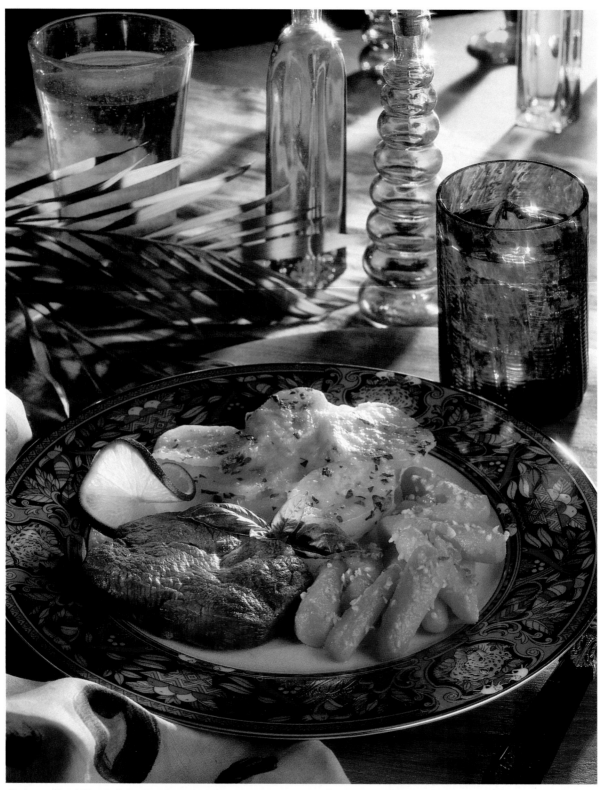

Calypso Beef Tenderloin Steak, Basil Scalloped Potatoes, and Coconut Baby Carrots (menu on page 94)

COMPANY DINNERS

*W*hether it's a promotion, an anniversary, or an "over-the-hill" celebration, you need a meal that's worthy of the occasion. Here are some menu ideas that will let you enjoy the party without abandoning your low-calorie program.

The Hearty V.I.P. Dinner (page 102), pictured on the cover, features tender pork medaillons with a flavorful mushroom gravy, rich-tasting potatoes, and steamed green beans. And for dessert, the menu suggests lime parfaits. They make the finale truly grand, tasting much richer than their 173 calories.

Both the veal and asparagus dishes in Easy and Elegant (page 99) are simple to prepare but well suited for guests. Turn to pages 130 through 135 to find a complementary dessert; Almond Biscotti or Refreshing Citrus Sorbet would be perfect.

Tropical Dining
(pictured on page 92)

Servings		*Calories*
1 serving	Calypso Beef Tenderloin Steaks	233
1 serving	Coconut Baby Carrots	105
1 serving	Basil Scalloped Potatoes	161
1 serving	Lemon-Sauced Cakes	155
1 cup	Apple juice spritzer	58

———

Serves 6
Total Calories per Serving: 712
(Calories from Fat: 26%)

Calypso Beef Tenderloin Steaks

¾ cup canned low-sodium chicken broth
½ cup unsweetened orange juice
2½ tablespoons reduced-calorie ketchup
2 tablespoons brown sugar
2 tablespoons lime juice
2 tablespoons dark rum
1 teaspoon ground ginger
¼ teaspoon ground cloves
¼ teaspoon dried thyme
¼ teaspoon ground red pepper
1 large clove garlic, minced
1 (1½-pound) lean boneless beef tenderloin
Vegetable cooking spray
Lime slices (optional)
Fresh basil sprigs (optional)

Combine first 11 ingredients in a medium bowl; stir well with a wire whisk. Set marinade aside.

Trim fat from tenderloin; cut tenderloin crosswise into 6 equal steaks. Place in a large heavy-duty, zip-top plastic bag; pour marinade over steaks. Seal bag; shake well. Marinate in refrigerator 30 minutes, turning bag occasionally.

Remove steaks from marinade, reserving marinade. Place steaks on rack of a broiler pan coated with cooking spray. Broil 5½ inches from heat (with electric oven door partially opened) 6 to 8 minutes on each side or to desired degree of doneness, basting with reserved marinade. If desired, garnish with lime and basil. Yield: 6 servings.

Per Serving: 233 Calories (34% from Fat)
Fat 8.7g (Saturated Fat 3.3g)
Protein 25.9g   Carbohydrate 8.5g
Cholesterol 75mg   Sodium 71mg

Coconut Baby Carrots

1 (16-ounce) package frozen baby carrots, thawed
2 tablespoons reduced-calorie stick margarine
2 tablespoons honey
2 tablespoons chutney
½ teaspoon mustard seeds
¼ cup unsweetened grated coconut, toasted

Combine first 5 ingredients in a large skillet. Cook over medium-high heat until thoroughly heated, stirring occasionally. Transfer carrot mixture to a serving platter; sprinkle with coconut. Yield: 6 (½-cup) servings.

Per Serving: 105 Calories (36% from Fat)
Fat 4.2g (Saturated Fat 1.7g)
Protein 1.1g   Carbohydrate 17.7g
Cholesterol 0mg   Sodium 76mg

BASIL SCALLOPED POTATOES

Vegetable cooking spray
2 cloves garlic, minced
¾ cup skim milk, divided
1 tablespoon all-purpose flour
¾ cup evaporated skimmed milk
2 tablespoons chopped fresh basil
¼ teaspoon salt
¼ teaspoon dried crushed red pepper
⅛ teaspoon ground white pepper
4 cups peeled, thinly sliced baking potato
  (about 1¾ pounds)
½ cup (2 ounces) shredded Gruyère cheese
2 tablespoons freshly grated Parmesan cheese

Coat a large saucepan with cooking spray; place over medium-high heat until hot. Add garlic, and sauté until tender.

Combine ¼ cup skim milk and flour; stir with a wire whisk until smooth. Add flour mixture to garlic; cook, stirring constantly, 1 minute or until mixture thickens.

Gradually add remaining ½ cup skim milk, evaporated milk, and next 4 ingredients. Bring to a boil, stirring constantly. Add potato slices, and remove from heat.

Spoon half of potato mixture into an 11- x 7- x 1½-inch baking dish coated with cooking spray. Top with half of Gruyère cheese. Repeat layers. Sprinkle with Parmesan cheese.

Cover and bake at 350° for 30 minutes. Uncover and bake an additional 15 minutes. Let stand 10 minutes before serving. Yield: 6 (½-cup) servings.

PER SERVING: 161 CALORIES (23% FROM FAT)
FAT 4.1G (SATURATED FAT 2.3G)
PROTEIN 10.4G   CARBOHYDRATE 21.5G
CHOLESTEROL 14MG   SODIUM 232MG

LEMON-SAUCED CAKES

For a different flavor, use lime juice instead of lemon juice in the sauce.

¼ cup sugar
2 teaspoons cornstarch
Dash of salt
½ cup water
¾ teaspoon grated lemon rind
2½ tablespoons lemon juice
1 tablespoon margarine
8 ounces nonfat pound cake
¼ cup plus 2 tablespoons frozen reduced-
  calorie whipped topping, thawed

Combine sugar, cornstarch, and salt in a 2-cup glass measure. Add water; stir until sugar dissolves.

Microwave at HIGH 1 minute; stir well. Microwave at HIGH 1 to 1½ minutes, stirring at 30-second intervals, until mixture is clear, thickened, and bubbly.

Stir in lemon rind, lemon juice, and margarine.

Cut pound cake into 6 slices; place on individual serving plates. Top each slice with 2 tablespoons lemon sauce and 1 tablespoon whipped topping. Yield: 6 servings.

Note: Lemon sauce can be prepared on the stovetop. Combine sugar, cornstarch, and salt in a small saucepan; add water, stirring well. Place over medium heat, and cook, stirring constantly, until mixture is thickened and bubbly. Stir in lemon rind, lemon juice, and margarine.

PER SERVING: 155 CALORIES (20% FROM FAT)
FAT 3.5G (SATURATED FAT 0.7G)
PROTEIN 1.7G   CARBOHYDRATE 30.3G
CHOLESTEROL 0MG   SODIUM 184MG

Quick Tip

Mix equal amounts of chilled fruit juice with sparkling water for a refreshing fruit juice spritzer. Serve over ice with a sprig of mint or a slice of lime.

STEAK WITH A FLAIR

Servings		Calories
1 serving	Grilled Sirloin with Sweet Red Pepper Sauce	201
1 serving	Herbed Corn on the Cob	97
1 serving	Hot and Spicy Marinated Vegetables	29
1 slice	French bread	82
1 serving	Chocolate-Amaretto Pudding	188
6 ounces	Nonalcoholic red wine	48

Serves 4

TOTAL CALORIES PER SERVING: 645
(CALORIES FROM FAT: 20%)

GRILLED SIRLOIN WITH SWEET RED PEPPER SAUCE

1 (1-pound) lean boneless beef top sirloin steak
½ cup commercial fat-free Italian dressing
½ cup red wine vinegar
4 medium-size sweet red peppers, divided
⅓ cup chopped green onions
¼ cup water
2 tablespoons dry white wine
¾ teaspoon beef-flavored bouillon granules
Vegetable cooking spray

Trim fat from steak, and cut steak into 4 equal portions. Place in a large shallow dish. Combine dressing and vinegar; pour over steaks. Cover and marinate in refrigerator at least 8 hours, turning occasionally. Remove steaks from marinade; discard marinade.

Cut 1 pepper into thin strips; set aside. Seed and chop remaining peppers. Combine chopped pepper, green onions, and next 3 ingredients in a nonstick skillet; bring to a boil. Cover, reduce heat, and simmer 15 minutes. Cool slightly. Place chopped pepper mixture in container of an electric blender; cover and process until smooth. Strain mixture, and set aside.

Coat a grill rack with cooking spray; place on grill over medium-hot coals. Place steaks on rack, and grill 5 minutes on each side or to desired degree of doneness. Set aside; keep warm.

Coat skillet with cooking spray; place skillet over medium-high heat until hot. Add reserved pepper strips; sauté until tender. Remove from skillet; set aside. Add red pepper sauce to skillet; cook over low heat until thoroughly heated.

Place steaks on individual serving plates; spoon sauce evenly over steaks. Top evenly with pepper strips. Yield: 4 servings.

PER SERVING: 201 CALORIES (30% FROM FAT)
FAT 6.8G (SATURATED FAT 2.5G)
PROTEIN 26.7G   CARBOHYDRATE 6.9G
CHOLESTEROL 76MG   SODIUM 400MG

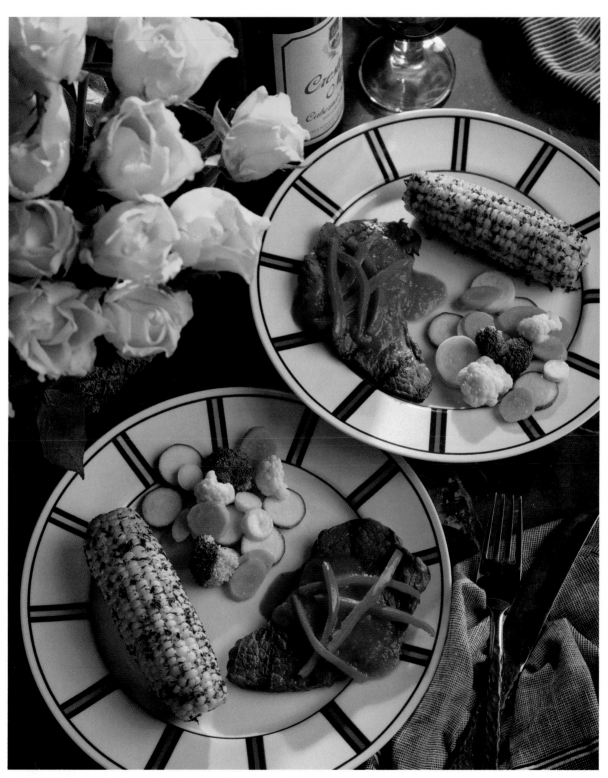

Grilled Sirloin with Sweet Red Pepper Sauce, Herbed Corn on the Cob, and Hot and Spicy Marinated Vegetables

HERBED CORN ON THE COB

4 ears fresh corn
1 tablespoon dried dillweed
1 tablespoon dried thyme
1 tablespoon water
1 teaspoon vegetable oil
1 clove garlic, minced

Remove husks and silk from corn; set aside.
Combine dillweed and next 4 ingredients in a small bowl, stirring well. Rub herb mixture evenly over corn; place each ear on a piece of heavy-duty aluminum foil. Roll foil lengthwise around each ear; twist foil at each end to seal.
Grill corn over medium-hot coals 15 to 20 minutes or until corn is tender, turning every 5 minutes. Yield: 4 servings.

PER SERVING: 97 CALORIES (20% FROM FAT)
FAT 2.2G (SATURATED FAT 0.4G)
PROTEIN 2.7G CARBOHYDRATE 20.2G
CHOLESTEROL 0MG SODIUM 15MG

HOT AND SPICY MARINATED VEGETABLES

½ cup fresh cauliflower flowerets
½ cup fresh broccoli flowerets
½ cup thinly sliced yellow squash
¼ cup thinly sliced zucchini
¼ cup diagonally sliced carrot
¼ cup white wine vinegar
½ teaspoon garlic powder
¾ teaspoon chili oil
½ teaspoon vegetable oil

Combine first 5 ingredients; set aside.
Combine vinegar, garlic powder, and oils; stir well. Pour vinegar mixture over vegetables; toss gently to coat. Cover and marinate in refrigerator at least 8 hours, tossing occasionally. Serve with a slotted spoon. Yield: 4 (½-cup) servings.
Note: Vegetable oil may be substituted for chili oil, if desired.

PER SERVING: 29 CALORIES (47% FROM FAT)
FAT 1.5G (SATURATED FAT 0.3G)
PROTEIN 1.0G CARBOHYDRATE 3.1G
CHOLESTEROL 0MG SODIUM 11MG

CHOCOLATE-AMARETTO PUDDING

If you prefer not to use amaretto, simply omit it from the recipe. You'll still get a smooth, rich-tasting chocolate pudding.

¼ cup plus 2 tablespoons sugar
3 tablespoons unsweetened cocoa
2 tablespoons plus 2 teaspoons cornstarch
2 cups 1% low-fat milk
2 teaspoons amaretto
½ teaspoon vanilla extract
1 tablespoon plus 1 teaspoon chopped almonds, toasted

Combine first 3 ingredients in a medium saucepan. Gradually add milk, stirring with a wire whisk until smooth. Cook over medium-low heat, stirring constantly, 10 minutes or until mixture is thickened. Remove from heat; stir in amaretto and vanilla.
Spoon mixture evenly into 4 dessert dishes. Cover and chill thoroughly. Just before serving, sprinkle evenly with almonds. Yield: 4 servings.

PER SERVING: 188 CALORIES (15% FROM FAT)
FAT 3.2G (SATURATED FAT 1.3G)
PROTEIN 5.7G CARBOHYDRATE 32.9G
CHOLESTEROL 5MG SODIUM 64MG

EASY AND ELEGANT

Servings		Calories
1 serving	Veal Cutlets in Peppercorn Sauce	194
1 serving	Asparagus Sauté	35
1 cup	Commercial saffron rice	258
1 slice	Italian bread	82

Serves 4
TOTAL CALORIES PER SERVING: 569
(CALORIES FROM FAT: 12%)

VEAL CUTLETS IN PEPPERCORN SAUCE

1 pound veal cutlets (¼ inch thick)
Vegetable cooking spray
1½ cups canned no-salt-added beef broth
½ cup dry red wine
1½ tablespoons green peppercorns, drained
½ teaspoon salt
2 large cloves garlic, crushed
2 bay leaves
1 tablespoon plus 1 teaspoon cornstarch
2 tablespoons water

Trim fat from cutlets. Coat a nonstick skillet with cooking spray; place over medium-high heat until hot. Add veal; cook 3 minutes on each side or until browned. Remove veal from skillet; drain and pat dry. Wipe drippings from skillet. Combine broth and next 5 ingredients in skillet; stir well. Add veal. Bring to a boil. Cover, reduce heat, and simmer 20 minutes or until veal is tender. Remove veal from skillet; set aside. Remove bay leaves.

Combine cornstarch and water; add to broth mixture. Cook, stirring constantly, until thickened. Return veal to skillet; cook until heated. Yield: 4 servings.

PER SERVING: 194 CALORIES (27% FROM FAT)
FAT 5.8G (SATURATED FAT 1.6G)
PROTEIN 27.7G CARBOHYDRATE 4.2G
CHOLESTEROL 100MG SODIUM 375MG

ASPARAGUS SAUTÉ

1 pound fresh asparagus spears
Vegetable cooking spray
1 clove garlic, minced
10 cherry tomatoes, halved
½ teaspoon dried oregano
⅛ teaspoon dried thyme
Dash of pepper
1 tablespoon grated Parmesan cheese

Snap off tough ends of asparagus spears. Remove scales from spears with a knife or vegetable peeler, if desired. Cut asparagus spears diagonally into 1-inch pieces. Arrange asparagus pieces in a vegetable steamer over boiling water. Cover and steam 4 to 5 minutes or until asparagus is crisp-tender.

Coat a large nonstick skillet with cooking spray; place over medium-high heat until hot. Add asparagus and garlic; sauté 4 to 5 minutes or until tender. Stir in tomato halves, oregano, thyme, and pepper. Cook 1 minute or until thoroughly heated, stirring constantly. Transfer mixture to a serving dish, and sprinkle evenly with Parmesan cheese. Yield: 4 (¾-cup) servings.

PER SERVING: 35 CALORIES (23% FROM FAT)
FAT 0.9G (SATURATED FAT 0.3G)
PROTEIN 2.6G CARBOHYDRATE 5.9G
CHOLESTEROL 1MG SODIUM 30MG

ENGLISH PUB SPECIAL

Servings		*Calories*
1 serving	Peppered Raspberry Lamb Chops	239
1 serving	Tarragon Brussels Sprouts	51
1 serving	Blue Cheese Potatoes	98
2 slices	Beer Bread	232
1 cup	Iced tea	2

Serves 2
TOTAL CALORIES PER SERVING: 622
(CALORIES FROM FAT: 19%)

PEPPERED RASPBERRY LAMB CHOPS

4 (4-ounce) lean lamb loin chops (1 inch thick)
½ teaspoon cracked pepper
Vegetable cooking spray
3 tablespoons low-sugar raspberry spread
2 teaspoons low-sodium Worcestershire sauce
1½ teaspoons raspberry-flavored vinegar
Fresh raspberries (optional)

Trim fat from chops. Press pepper into both sides of each chop. Place chops on rack of a broiler pan coated with cooking spray.

Broil 5½ inches from heat (with electric oven door partially opened) 6 to 7 minutes on each side or to desired degree of doneness. Transfer to a serving platter, and keep warm.

Combine raspberry spread, Worcestershire sauce, and vinegar in a saucepan; cook over medium heat until spread melts, stirring constantly. Spoon evenly over chops. Garnish with fresh raspberries, if desired. Yield: 2 servings.

PER SERVING: 239 CALORIES (33% FROM FAT)
FAT 8.7G (SATURATED FAT 3.0G)
PROTEIN 26.3G   CARBOHYDRATE 12.5G
CHOLESTEROL 83MG   SODIUM 117MG

TARRAGON BRUSSELS SPROUTS

If you don't have fresh tarragon, use ⅛ to ¼ teaspoon of dried tarragon.

1 cup small fresh brussels sprouts (about ¼ pound)
2 tablespoons chopped onion
½ teaspoon minced fresh tarragon
½ cup canned low-sodium chicken broth, undiluted
1½ teaspoons reduced-calorie margarine, melted

Wash brussels sprouts thoroughly, and remove discolored leaves. Cut off stem ends, and cut a shallow X in bottom of each sprout.

Combine brussels sprouts, onion, tarragon, and chicken broth in a medium saucepan; bring to a boil. Cover, reduce heat, and simmer 10 to 12 minutes or until brussels sprouts are tender. Drain well. Drizzle margarine over brussels sprouts, and toss gently. Yield: 2 (½-cup) servings.

PER SERVING: 51 CALORIES (35% FROM FAT)
FAT 2.0G (SATURATED FAT 0.3G)
PROTEIN 2.2G   CARBOHYDRATE 6.9G
CHOLESTEROL 0MG   SODIUM 43MG

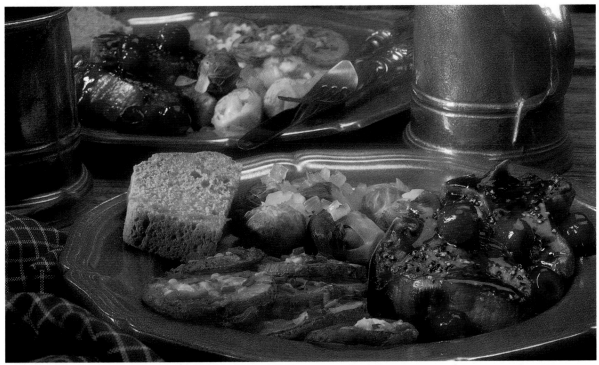

Peppered Raspberry Lamb Chops, Blue Cheese Potatoes, Beer Bread, and Tarragon Brussels Sprouts

BLUE CHEESE POTATOES

Butter-flavored vegetable cooking spray
1 medium baking potato, cut into ¼-inch slices
¼ cup chopped green pepper
¼ cup chopped onion
1 tablespoon crumbled blue cheese
2 teaspoons minced fresh chives

Coat a large nonstick skillet with cooking spray; place over medium-high heat until hot. Add potato; cook 7 to 8 minutes or until browned, turning occasionally. Add green pepper and onion. Cover, reduce heat, and cook 20 minutes or until tender, turning occasionally. Sprinkle with cheese; cover and cook 1 minute or until cheese melts. Sprinkle with chives, and serve immediately. Yield: 2 (½-cup) servings.

PER SERVING: 98 CALORIES (13% FROM FAT)
FAT 1.4G (SATURATED FAT 0.7G)
PROTEIN 3.3G   CARBOHYDRATE 18.8G
CHOLESTEROL 3MG   SODIUM 57MG

BEER BREAD

2 cups all-purpose flour
1½ cups whole wheat flour
1 tablespoon baking powder
½ teaspoon salt
3 tablespoons brown sugar
2 teaspoons caraway seeds
3 tablespoons golden raisins, chopped
1 (12-ounce) can light beer, at room temperature
¼ cup frozen egg substitute, thawed
Vegetable cooking spray

Combine first 7 ingredients. Add beer and egg substitute, stirring until dry ingredients are moistened. Spoon into an 8½- x 4½- x 3-inch loafpan coated with cooking spray. Bake at 375° for 45 minutes or until a wooden pick inserted in center comes out clean. Cool in pan 10 minutes. Remove from pan; cool on a wire rack. Yield: 16 (½-inch) slices.

PER SLICE: 116 CALORIES (3% FROM FAT)
FAT 0.4G (SATURATED FAT 0.1G)
PROTEIN 3.6G   CARBOHYDRATE 23.8G
CHOLESTEROL 0MG   SODIUM 138MG

HEARTY V.I.P. DINNER

(pictured on cover)

Servings		*Calories*
1 serving	Pork Madeira	155
½ cup	Steamed green beans	22
1 serving	Mashed Potatoes	119
1 roll	French roll	164
1 serving	Key West Lime Parfaits	173

Serves 4

TOTAL CALORIES PER SERVING: 633
(CALORIES FROM FAT: 15%)

PORK MADEIRA

1 pound pork tenderloin, cut into ½-inch-thick
   slices
¼ teaspoon pepper
Vegetable cooking spray
1 cup thinly sliced fresh mushrooms
1 cup water
¼ cup Madeira
2 teaspoons low-sodium Worcestershire sauce
1 teaspoon beef-flavored bouillon granules
2 tablespoons cornstarch
2 tablespoons water
1 tablespoon plus 1 teaspoon minced fresh
   chives

Sprinkle pork with pepper. Coat a large nonstick skillet with cooking spray; place skillet over medium heat until hot. Add pork, and cook 4 minutes on each side or until browned. Remove pork, and drain on paper towels. Wipe skillet dry with a paper towel.

Coat skillet with cooking spray; place over medium heat until hot. Add mushrooms; sauté 2 minutes or until tender. Add 1 cup water and next 3 ingredients; bring to a boil, and cook, stirring constantly, until some of liquid evaporates.

Combine cornstarch and 2 tablespoons water, stirring well; stir into mushroom mixture in skillet. Cook over medium heat, stirring constantly, until mixture comes to a full boil. Boil 1 minute, stirring constantly. Add pork and chives to skillet, and cook over medium heat until thoroughly heated. Spoon gravy over pork and potatoes, if desired. Yield: 4 servings.

PER SERVING: 155 CALORIES (19% FROM FAT)
FAT 3.2G (SATURATED FAT 1.1G)
PROTEIN 24.2G CARBOHYDRATE 5.4G
CHOLESTEROL 74MG SODIUM 303MG

MASHED POTATOES

4 medium baking potatoes, peeled and cut into
   ½-inch pieces (about 1½ pounds)
¼ cup nonfat sour cream
2 tablespoons evaporated skimmed milk
¼ teaspoon salt
Dash of ground white pepper
½ teaspoon margarine

Place potato in a saucepan; add water to cover, and bring to a boil. Cover, reduce heat, and simmer 20 minutes or until very tender; drain. Combine potato, sour cream, and next 4 ingredients in a bowl; beat at medium speed of an electric mixer 2 minutes or until smooth. Yield: 4 (¾-cup) servings.

PER SERVING: 119 CALORIES (5% FROM FAT)
FAT 0.7G (SATURATED FAT 0.1G)
PROTEIN 6.0G CARBOHYDRATE 23.1G
CHOLESTEROL 0MG SODIUM 188MG

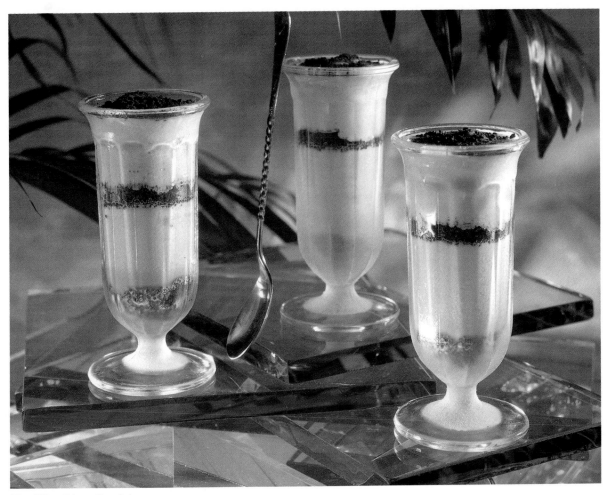

Key West Lime Parfaits

KEY WEST LIME PARFAITS

Vegetable cooking spray
2 tablespoons finely chopped unsalted
    macadamia nuts
⅓ cup chocolate wafer cookie crumbs
2 cups lime sherbet, softened
2 teaspoons grated lime rind
1 tablespoon plus 1 teaspoon chocolate wafer
    cookie crumbs

Coat a 1-quart baking dish with cooking spray. Spread nuts in baking dish, and microwave, uncovered, at HIGH 4 to 6 minutes or until lightly toasted, stirring every 30 seconds. Combine toasted nuts and ⅓ cup chocolate wafer cookie crumbs; stir well, and set cookie crumb mixture aside.

Combine lime sherbet and lime rind in a medium bowl; stir well.

Spoon 1 tablespoon chocolate cookie crumb mixture into each of 4 (6-ounce) parfait glasses; top each with ¼ cup sherbet mixture. Spoon 1 tablespoon crumb mixture over each; top each with ¼ cup sherbet mixture. Sprinkle each serving with 1 teaspoon cookie crumbs. Cover and freeze until firm. Yield: 4 servings.

PER SERVING: 173 CALORIES (30% FROM FAT)
FAT 5.7G (SATURATED FAT 1.4G)
PROTEIN 1.8G CARBOHYDRATE 29.9G
CHOLESTEROL 7MG SODIUM 103MG

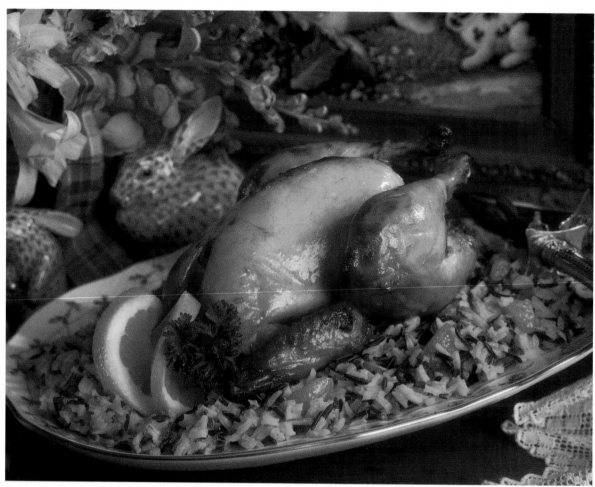

Oriental Chicken and Orange-Almond Rice

SPECIAL OCCASION MENU

Servings		*Calories*
1 serving	Oriental Chicken	167
1 serving	Orange-Almond Rice	264
1 serving	Roasted Asparagus with Onions	37
2 muffins	Miniature Carrot Cake Muffins	94
1 serving	Frozen Lemon Angel Cake	134

Serves 6

TOTAL CALORIES PER SERVING: 696
(CALORIES FROM FAT: 18%)

ORIENTAL CHICKEN

1 (3-pound) broiler-fryer, skinned
2 cups dry sherry
½ cup white wine vinegar
½ cup low-sodium teriyaki sauce
⅓ cup firmly packed brown sugar
5 cloves garlic, minced
Vegetable cooking spray
Orange slices (optional)
Fresh parsley sprigs (optional)

Trim fat from chicken. Remove giblets and neck; reserve for another use. Rinse chicken under cold water; pat dry with paper towels. Combine sherry and next 4 ingredients; cover and chill ½ cup sherry mixture. Place remaining sherry mixture in a large heavy-duty, zip-top bag; add chicken. Seal bag; shake until chicken is coated. Marinate in refrigerator 8 hours, turning bag occasionally.

Remove chicken from marinade; discard marinade. Place chicken, breast side up, on a rack in a roasting pan coated with cooking spray. Insert meat thermometer into meaty part of thigh, making sure it does not touch bone. Cover and bake at 400° for 40 minutes; uncover and bake 30 minutes or until meat thermometer registers 180°, basting occasionally with ½ cup sherry mixture. If desired, garnish with orange slices and parsley. Yield: 6 servings.

PER SERVING: 167 CALORIES (33% FROM FAT)
FAT 6.2G (SATURATED FAT 1.7G)
PROTEIN 23.8G CARBOHYDRATE 2.5G
CHOLESTEROL 73MG SODIUM 118MG

ORANGE-ALMOND RICE

2½ cups canned no-salt-added chicken broth
1½ cups unsweetened orange juice
¼ teaspoon salt
¾ cup wild rice, uncooked
¼ cup chopped onion
1 cup long-grain rice, uncooked
⅓ cup canned mandarin oranges in light
    syrup, drained
¼ cup sliced almonds, toasted
2 tablespoons chopped fresh parsley
¼ teaspoon pepper

Combine chicken broth, unsweetened orange juice, and salt in a medium saucepan; bring mixture to a boil.

Add wild rice and chopped onion to mixture in saucepan; cover, reduce heat, and simmer 20 minutes. Add long-grain rice; cover and simmer an additional 30 minutes or until rice is tender and liquid is absorbed.

Add oranges, almonds, parsley, and pepper to rice mixture in saucepan; stir well. Yield: 6 (1-cup) servings.

PER SERVING: 264 CALORIES (10% FROM FAT)
FAT 2.9G (SATURATED FAT 0.3G)
PROTEIN 6.8G CARBOHYDRATE 51.7G
CHOLESTEROL 0MG SODIUM 105MG

ROASTED ASPARAGUS WITH ONIONS

1 pound fresh asparagus spears
1 large purple onion, thinly sliced
Vegetable cooking spray
2 tablespoons balsamic vinegar
1½ teaspoons grated orange rind
2 tablespoons fresh orange juice
1 teaspoon dark sesame oil
½ teaspoon freshly ground pepper
¼ teaspoon salt
¼ teaspoon sugar

Snap off tough ends of asparagus. Remove scales from stalks with a knife or vegetable peeler, if desired. Arrange asparagus and onion separately on 2 baking sheets coated with cooking spray. Bake onion at 400° for 15 to 18 minutes or until lightly browned, stirring twice. Bake asparagus at 400° for 12 to 15 minutes or until crisp-tender.

Combine vinegar and next 6 ingredients in a small jar; cover tightly and shake vigorously. Arrange asparagus and onion on a serving platter. Drizzle vinegar mixture over vegetables. Serve warm or at room temperature. Yield: 6 servings.

PER SERVING: 37 CALORIES (27% FROM FAT)
FAT 1.1G (SATURATED FAT 0.1G)
PROTEIN 1.6G CARBOHYDRATE 6.4G
CHOLESTEROL 0MG SODIUM 100MG

MINIATURE CARROT CAKE MUFFINS

1¼ cups sifted cake flour
1 teaspoon baking powder
¾ teaspoon baking soda
¼ teaspoon salt
½ teaspoon ground cinnamon
⅔ cup sugar
3 egg whites, lightly beaten
¼ cup apple butter
1 tablespoon vegetable oil
¾ cup grated carrot
⅓ cup canned crushed pineapple in juice, drained
Vegetable cooking spray

Combine first 6 ingredients in a medium bowl; make a well in center of mixture. Combine egg whites, apple butter, and oil; add to dry ingredients, stirring just until dry ingredients are moistened. Gently fold in carrot and pineapple.

Spoon batter into miniature (1¾-inch) muffin pans coated with cooking spray, filling three-fourths full. Bake at 375° for 13 minutes or until golden. Remove from pans immediately. Yield: 2½ dozen.

PER MUFFIN: 47 CALORIES (12% FROM FAT)
FAT 0.6G (SATURATED FAT 0.1G)
PROTEIN 0.7G CARBOHYDRATE 9.7G
CHOLESTEROL 0MG SODIUM 57MG

FROZEN LEMON ANGEL CAKE

You can replace the lemon ice cream called for in this dessert with your favorite flavor of low-fat ice cream, frozen yogurt, or sherbet.

1 (10½-ounce) loaf commercial angel food cake
1½ cups lemon low-fat ice cream, softened
1 (10-ounce) package frozen sliced strawberries in light syrup, thawed and drained
1¼ cups frozen reduced-calorie whipped topping, thawed
Fresh strawberries (optional)
Lemon slices (optional)
Fresh mint sprigs (optional)

Cut a ½-inch slice off top of cake; set aside. Hollow out center of cake, leaving a ½-inch-thick shell. Reserve inside of cake for another use. Combine ice milk and sliced strawberries, stirring well. Spoon ice milk mixture into cake shell; top with reserved cake slice. Cover and freeze 4 hours or until firm.

Place cake on a serving platter; spread whipped topping evenly over top and sides of cake. If desired, garnish with fresh strawberries, lemon slices, and mint sprigs. Serve immediately. Yield: 10 servings.

PER SERVING: 134 CALORIES (16% FROM FAT)
FAT 2.4G (SATURATED FAT 1.5G)
PROTEIN 2.8G CARBOHYDRATE 26.3G
CHOLESTEROL 4MG SODIUM 67MG

Menu Timetable

Early in the day, make the muffins and the dessert (to be covered with whipped topping just before serving). If you have enough room in the oven, roast the asparagus and onions while the chicken bakes. Just put the vegetables in the oven 15 to 30 minutes before the chicken is done. The vegetables are also delicious served at room temperature and may be baked earlier, if needed. While the chicken bakes, you can prepare the rice.

RESPITE AFTER WORK

Servings		Calories
1 serving	Chicken Breast Dijon	192
1 cup	Steamed Sugar Snap peas	67
1 serving	Brown Rice Pilaf	186
1 cup	Fresh fruit cup	100
	(equal amounts of grapes, orange sections, and pear slices)	

Serves 4
TOTAL CALORIES PER SERVING: 545
(CALORIES FROM FAT: 12%)

CHICKEN BREAST DIJON

⅓ cup fine, dry breadcrumbs
1 tablespoon Parmesan cheese
1 teaspoon dried Italian seasoning
½ teaspoon dried thyme
¼ teaspoon salt
¼ teaspoon freshly ground pepper
4 (4-ounce) skinned, boned chicken breast
   halves
2 tablespoons Dijon mustard
1 teaspoon olive oil
1 teaspoon reduced-calorie margarine

Combine first 6 ingredients in a small bowl, stirring well. Brush both sides of each chicken breast half with mustard; dredge in breadcrumb mixture.

Heat olive oil and margarine in a nonstick skillet over medium-high heat until margarine melts. Add chicken breasts, and cook 6 to 8 minutes on each side or until chicken is done. Yield: 4 servings.

PER SERVING: 192 CALORIES (22% FROM FAT)
FAT 4.6G (SATURATED FAT 1.0G)
PROTEIN 27.9G   CARBOHYDRATE 7.5G
CHOLESTEROL 67MG   SODIUM 553MG

BROWN RICE PILAF

½ cup diced carrot
½ cup diced sweet red pepper
1 cup brown rice, uncooked
3 cups water
½ teaspoon salt
½ teaspoon dried oregano
½ teaspoon dried thyme
2 large cloves garlic, minced

Arrange carrot and red pepper in a vegetable steamer over boiling water. Cover and steam 2 to 3 minutes or until vegetables are crisp-tender. Drain well, and set aside.

Combine rice and next 5 ingredients in a large saucepan. Bring to a boil; cover, reduce heat, and simmer 45 minutes.

Add vegetable mixture to rice mixture; toss gently. Cover and cook an additional 5 minutes or until rice is tender and liquid is absorbed. Yield: 4 (1-cup) servings.

PER SERVING: 186 CALORIES (7% FROM FAT)
FAT 1.4G (SATURATED FAT 0.4G)
PROTEIN 4.2G   CARBOHYDRATE 39.2G
CHOLESTEROL 0MG   SODIUM 304MG

MAKE-AHEAD DINNER

Servings		Calories
1 cup	Club soda with lime	0
1 serving	Roasted Coq au Vin and Vegetables	289
1 serving	Tossed Salad Supremo	57
1 slice	French bread	82
1 serving	Orange Amaretti	168

Serves 6
TOTAL CALORIES PER SERVING: 596
(CALORIES FROM FAT: 23%)

ROASTED COQ AU VIN AND VEGETABLES

Skin the chicken a day ahead, and prepare the vegetables early in the day. Use a turkey baster to baste chicken and vegetables with juices from the bottom of the pan.

⅓ cup all-purpose flour
1 teaspoon paprika
½ teaspoon salt
½ teaspoon freshly ground pepper
3 chicken breast halves, skinned (about 1½ pounds)
3 chicken thighs, skinned (about 1 pound)
3 chicken drumsticks, skinned (about ¾ pound)
1 tablespoon olive oil, divided
1 cup canned low-sodium chicken broth, undiluted
½ cup dry, white vermouth
1 teaspoon dried thyme
1 teaspoon dried rosemary
¼ pound small shallots (about 12), peeled
8 cloves garlic, peeled
1 (16-ounce) package fresh whole baby carrots
¾ pound unpeeled small round red potatoes (about 6), quartered
1 (8-ounce) package fresh crimini or button mushrooms, stems removed
¼ teaspoon salt

Combine first 4 ingredients in a large heavy-duty, zip-top plastic bag. Add chicken pieces to bag; seal bag, and toss to coat.

Heat 1½ teaspoons oil in a large nonstick skillet over medium heat. Add half of chicken pieces, shaking off excess flour. Cook 5 minutes on each side or until browned. Remove chicken from skillet; place in a shallow roasting pan. Repeat procedure with remaining oil and chicken; set aside.

Add broth and next 5 ingredients to skillet, and cook over medium heat 1 minute. Remove from heat, and set aside.

Arrange carrots, potato, and mushrooms around chicken in roasting pan. Pour broth mixture over chicken and vegetables; sprinkle vegetables with ¼ teaspoon salt. Bake, uncovered, at 400° for 1 hour and 5 minutes or until chicken is done and vegetables are tender, basting occasionally with juices in pan. Yield: 6 servings.

PER SERVING: 289 CALORIES (19% FROM FAT)
FAT 6.2G (SATURATED FAT 1.2G)
PROTEIN 29.0G   CARBOHYDRATE 29.5G
CHOLESTEROL 78MG   SODIUM 428MG

Tossed Salad Supremo

Make the salad and dressing up to 4 hours before dinner, chilling them in separate containers.

6 cups tightly packed bitter greens
1/3 cup (1¼ ounces) crumbled feta cheese
1/4 cup chopped fresh basil
3 plum tomatoes, quartered lengthwise
3 tablespoons canned low-sodium chicken
    broth, undiluted
2 tablespoons balsamic vinegar
1½ teaspoons olive oil
1/4 teaspoon sugar
1/4 teaspoon salt
1/4 teaspoon freshly ground pepper
1 clove garlic, minced

Combine first 4 ingredients in a large bowl, and toss gently.

Combine broth and next 6 ingredients; stir well. Pour over greens mixture just before serving, and toss gently. Yield: 6 servings.

Note: Bitter greens may be available premixed in your supermarket. If not, combine arugula, curly endive, radicchio, and watercress.

PER SERVING: 57 CALORIES (46% FROM FAT)
FAT 2.9G (SATURATED FAT 1.1G)
PROTEIN 3.2G CARBOHYDRATE 5.7G
CHOLESTEROL 5MG SODIUM 182MG

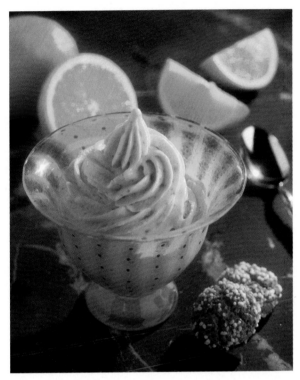

Orange Amaretti

Orange Amaretti

Pipe the sherbet mixture into dessert dishes, and freeze until serving time.

¾ cup frozen reduced-calorie whipped topping,
    thawed
3 amaretti cookies, crushed
2¼ cups orange sherbet, softened
6 amaretti cookies

Fold whipped topping and crushed cookies into sherbet. Pipe or spoon into dessert dishes. Serve each with 1 amaretti cookie. Serve immediately. Yield: 6 servings.

PER SERVING: 168 CALORIES (28% FROM FAT)
FAT 5.3G (SATURATED FAT 2.4G)
PROTEIN 1.6G CARBOHYDRATE 30.5G
CHOLESTEROL 4MG SODIUM 92MG

Focus on Fitness

Don't underestimate the benefits of stretching. It's a simple activity that promotes flexibility, prevents injuries, and makes you feel good. Here's what to remember:
• Try to stretch every day.
• Warm up your muscles with some simple fluid movements before you start to stretch.
• Concentrate on all major muscle groups.
• Hold each stretch for 30 to 60 seconds.

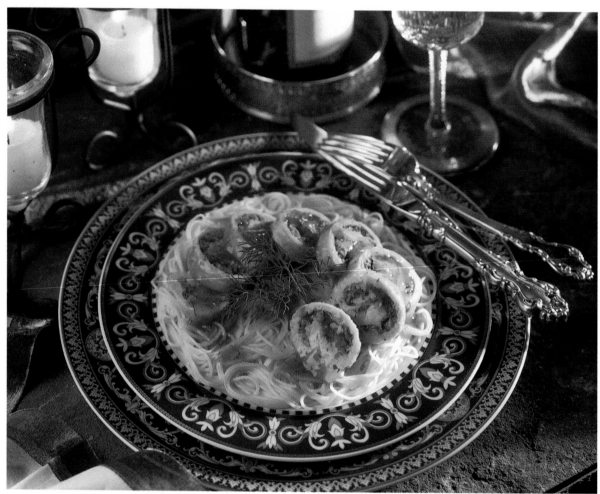

Stuffed Turkey Rolls and Pasta

CELEBRATION DINNER

Servings		*Calories*
1 serving	Stuffed Turkey Rolls and Pasta	288
1½ cups	Spinach salad with fat-free Italian dressing	23
2 rolls	Whole Wheat Cloverleaf Rolls	256
¾ cup	Sparkling white grape juice	36

Serves 4

TOTAL CALORIES PER SERVING: 603
(CALORIES FROM FAT: 15%)

STUFFED TURKEY ROLLS AND PASTA

½ cup frozen artichoke hearts, thawed and finely chopped
¼ cup finely chopped fresh mushrooms
¼ cup (1 ounce) shredded reduced-fat Swiss cheese
2 tablespoons finely chopped sweet red pepper
4 (4-ounce) turkey breast cutlets
Vegetable cooking spray
¾ cup plus 2 tablespoons canned no-salt-added chicken broth, undiluted and divided
¼ cup dry white wine
½ teaspoon dried dillweed
¼ teaspoon salt
1 tablespoon cornstarch
4 ounces capellini (angel hair pasta), uncooked
Fresh dill sprigs (optional)

Combine first 4 ingredients; stir and set aside.

Place turkey cutlets between 2 sheets of heavy-duty plastic wrap; flatten to ¼-inch thickness, using a meat mallet or rolling pin. Spoon artichoke mixture evenly onto centers of turkey cutlets. Roll up cutlets lengthwise, tucking ends under. Secure cutlets with wooden picks.

Coat a nonstick skillet with cooking spray; place over medium-high heat until hot. Add turkey rolls; cook until browned on all sides. Add ¾ cup broth, wine, dillweed, and salt; cover and cook 10 minutes or until turkey is tender. Remove turkey from skillet, using a slotted spoon; set aside, and keep warm.

Combine cornstarch and remaining 2 tablespoons broth. Add cornstarch mixture to liquid in skillet, stirring constantly. Bring to a boil over medium heat; cook, stirring constantly, 1 minute.

Cook pasta according to package directions, omitting salt and fat; drain. Divide pasta among 4 plates. Remove picks from turkey rolls. Cut each roll into 8 (¼-inch-thick) slices; arrange over pasta, and drizzle with sauce. Garnish with dill sprigs, if desired. Yield: 4 servings.

PER SERVING: 288 CALORIES (12% FROM FAT)
FAT 3.8G (SATURATED FAT 1.4G)
PROTEIN 33.9G   CARBOHYDRATE 27.0G
CHOLESTEROL 72MG   SODIUM 249MG

WHOLE WHEAT CLOVERLEAF ROLLS

2 tablespoons sugar, divided
1 package active dry yeast
¼ cup warm water (105° to 115°)
1½ cups all-purpose flour, divided
1 cup whole wheat flour
½ teaspoon salt
¼ cup warm 1% low-fat milk (105° to 115°)
1 tablespoon vegetable oil
1 egg
Vegetable cooking spray
1 tablespoon margarine, melted

Dissolve 1 teaspoon sugar and yeast in warm water, and let stand 5 minutes. Place remaining 1 tablespoon plus 2 teaspoons sugar, 1¼ cups all-purpose flour, whole wheat flour, and salt in food processor, and pulse 2 times. With food processor on, add yeast mixture, milk, oil, and egg through food chute; process until dough leaves sides of bowl and forms a ball. Process an additional 1 minute (dough will be sticky).

Turn dough out onto a lightly floured surface. Knead until smooth and elastic (about 5 minutes); add enough of remaining flour, 1 tablespoon at a time, to prevent dough from sticking to hands. Place dough in a large bowl coated with cooking spray, turning to coat top. Cover and let rise in a warm place (85°), free from drafts, 1 hour or until doubled in bulk. Punch dough down; cover and let rest 5 minutes.

Coat 12 muffin cups with cooking spray. Divide dough into 12 equal portions. Divide each portion into 3 pieces; shape each piece into a ball. Dip balls in melted margarine; place 3 balls in each muffin cup. Cover and let rise 45 minutes or until doubled in bulk. Uncover dough; bake at 400° for 15 minutes or until browned. Remove from pans, and serve warm. Yield: 1 dozen.

PER ROLL: 128 CALORIES (21% FROM FAT)
FAT 3.0G (SATURATED FAT 0.6G)
PROTEIN 3.9G   CARBOHYDRATE 21.8G
CHOLESTEROL 19MG   SODIUM 118MG

FRENCH FARE

Servings		_Calories_
1 serving	Grilled Amberjack au Poivre	134
1 serving	Tangy Carrot-Jicama Salad	59
1 roll	Sourdough rolls	160
1 serving	Peaches en Papillote with Raspberry Sauce	59

Serves 6
TOTAL CALORIES PER SERVING: 412
(CALORIES FROM FAT: 13%)

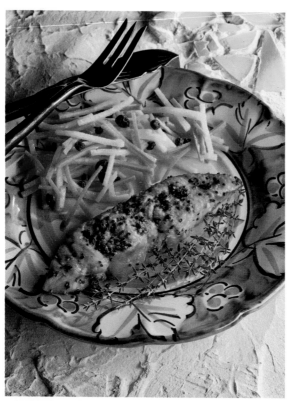

Grilled Amberjack au Poivre and Tangy Carrot-Jicama Salad

GRILLED AMBERJACK AU POIVRE

6 (4-ounce) amberjack steaks
⅓ cup lemon juice
⅓ cup red wine vinegar
1 tablespoon sugar
1 teaspoon minced fresh thyme
⅛ teaspoon salt
3 cloves garlic, minced
3 tablespoons cracked pepper
Vegetable cooking spray
Fresh thyme sprigs (optional)

Place amberjack in a shallow dish. Combine lemon juice and next 5 ingredients in a small bowl; stir well. Pour over fish, turning to coat. Cover and marinate in refrigerator 30 minutes, turning occasionally.

Remove fish from marinade, discarding marinade. Sprinkle pepper evenly over both sides of fish, pressing pepper into fish.

Coat grill rack with cooking spray. Place on grill over medium coals (300° to 350°). Place fish on rack; grill, covered, 4 to 6 minutes on each side or until fish flakes easily when tested with a fork. (Do not overcook or the fish will be dry.) Garnish with thyme sprigs, if desired. Yield: 6 servings.

PER SERVING: 134 CALORIES (16% FROM FAT)
FAT 2.4G (SATURATED FAT 0.6G)
PROTEIN 21.4G   CARBOHYDRATE 6.3G
CHOLESTEROL 47MG   SODIUM 126MG

TANGY CARROT-JICAMA SALAD

½ cup unsweetened orange juice
3 tablespoons white wine vinegar
1 tablespoon plus 1 teaspoon vegetable oil
¼ teaspoon salt
⅛ teaspoon freshly ground pepper
2 large carrots, scraped and cut into thin strips
½ small jicama, peeled and cut into thin strips
3 tablespoons currants

Combine first 5 ingredients in a shallow dish; stir with a wire whisk until well blended.

Add carrot, jicama, and currants; toss gently to coat. Cover and chill at least 30 minutes, tossing occasionally. Serve with a slotted spoon. Yield: 6 (½-cup) servings.

PER SERVING: 59 CALORIES (26% FROM FAT)
FAT 1.7G (SATURATED FAT 0.3G)
PROTEIN 0.8G   CARBOHYDRATE 10.6G
CHOLESTEROL 0MG   SODIUM 62MG

PEACHES EN PAPILLOTE WITH RASPBERRY SAUCE

1 (16-ounce) bag frozen sliced unsweetened peaches, thawed
Raspberry Sauce

Cut 6 (10-inch) squares of parchment paper; fold squares in half, creasing firmly. Trim each folded rectangle into a large heart shape.

Arrange 5 peach slices on a paper heart near the crease. Fold over remaining half of heart. Starting with rounded edge, pleat and crimp edges together to make a seal. Twist end tightly to seal; place on a large baking sheet. Repeat with remaining peach slices and paper hearts.

Bake peaches at 425° for 12 minutes or until parchment bags are puffed and lightly browned. Place bags on individual dessert plates, and cut open. Spoon warm Raspberry Sauce evenly over peaches, and serve warm. Yield: 6 servings.

RASPBERRY SAUCE

1 cup frozen unsweetened raspberries, thawed
3 tablespoons water
1½ teaspoons cornstarch
1½ tablespoons raspberry or other fruit-flavored schnapps
2 teaspoons sugar

Place raspberries in container of an electric blender; cover and process until smooth. Place raspberry puree in a wire-mesh strainer; press with back of spoon against the sides of the strainer to squeeze out ½ cup puree. Discard seeds and pulp in strainer.

Combine raspberry puree, water, and cornstarch in a saucepan; stir well. Add schnapps and sugar; cook over medium heat, stirring constantly, until thickened and bubbly. Serve warm. Yield: ⅔ cup.

PER SERVING: 59 CALORIES (3% FROM FAT)
FAT 0.2G (SATURATED FAT 0.0G)
PROTEIN 0.7G   CARBOHYDRATE 14.8G
CHOLESTEROL 0MG   SODIUM 0MG

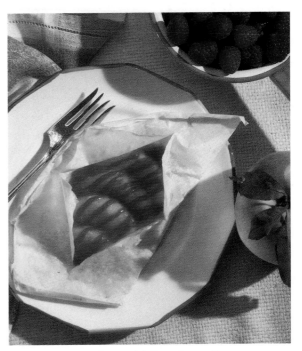

Peaches en Papillote with Raspberry Sauce

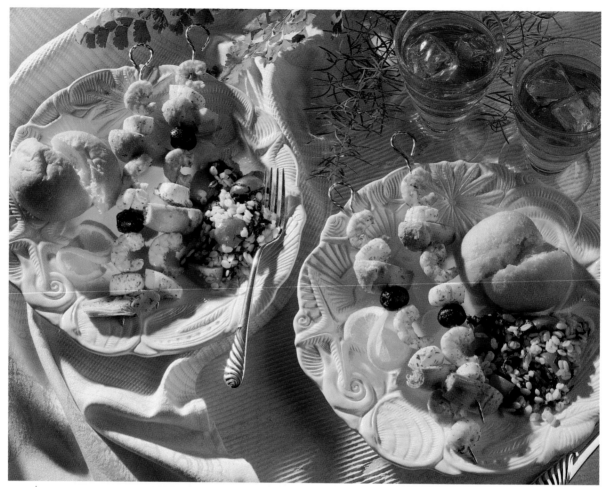

Shrimp and Scallop Kabobs and Spinach-Laced Barley

DINNER FOR TWO

Servings		*Calories*
1 serving	Shrimp and Scallop Kabobs	145
1 serving	Spinach-Laced Barley	86
1 roll	Commercial dinner rolls	127
1 serving	Lemon Sorbet with Summer Fruits	199
1 cup	Iced tea	2

Serves 2

TOTAL CALORIES PER SERVING: 559
(CALORIES FROM FAT: 14%)

SHRIMP AND SCALLOP KABOBS

This elegant entrée marinates and cooks in less than 30 minutes.

½ cup dry white wine
2 tablespoons lemon juice
1 tablespoon Creole mustard
1 teaspoon vegetable oil
¼ teaspoon dried dillweed
⅛ teaspoon hot sauce
¼ pound fresh sea scallops
¼ pound medium-size fresh shrimp, peeled
    and deveined
4 frozen artichoke hearts, thawed and halved
4 pitted ripe olives
Vegetable cooking spray

Combine first 6 ingredients in a dish. Add scallops, shrimp, and artichoke hearts to wine mixture; toss. Cover and marinate in refrigerator 15 minutes.

Remove scallops, shrimp, and artichokes from marinade, reserving marinade; place marinade in a saucepan. Bring to a boil over medium-high heat; boil 2 minutes. Remove from heat; set aside.

Thread scallops, shrimp, artichokes, and olives alternately on 4 (10-inch) skewers. Place kabobs on rack of a broiler pan coated with cooking spray. Broil 5½ inches from heat (with electric oven door partially opened) 6 minutes or until scallops are opaque and shrimp are done, turning once and basting with reserved marinade. Yield: 2 servings.

PER SERVING: 145 CALORIES (30% FROM FAT)
FAT 4.9G (SATURATED FAT 0.8G)
PROTEIN 16.6G CARBOHYDRATE 10.7G
CHOLESTEROL 75MG SODIUM 395MG

SPINACH-LACED BARLEY

½ cup water
3 tablespoons quick-cooking barley, uncooked
Vegetable cooking spray
2 tablespoons minced onion
1 clove garlic, minced
1 cup thinly sliced fresh spinach leaves
2 cherry tomatoes, quartered
⅛ teaspoon salt
Dash of pepper

Bring water to a boil in a saucepan; add barley. Cover, reduce heat, and simmer 10 to 12 minutes or until barley is tender. Remove from heat; let stand 5 minutes.

Coat a small nonstick skillet with cooking spray; place over medium-high heat until hot. Add onion and garlic; sauté until tender. Stir in cooked barley, spinach, tomatoes, salt, and pepper. Cook 1 to 3 minutes or until spinach wilts and tomatoes are thoroughly heated. Yield: 2 (½-cup) servings.

PER SERVING: 86 CALORIES (9% FROM FAT)
FAT 0.9G (SATURATED FAT 0.1G)
PROTEIN 3.4G CARBOHYDRATE 17.4G
CHOLESTEROL 0MG SODIUM 173MG

LEMON SORBET WITH SUMMER FRUITS

2 fresh apricots, seeded and quartered
½ cup fresh raspberries
½ cup chopped fresh pineapple
½ cup cubed honeydew melon
1 cup lemon sorbet or sherbet

Arrange fruits on 2 individual dessert plates or in shallow bowls. Scoop ½ cup sorbet onto each serving of fruit; serve immediately. Yield: 2 servings.

PER SERVING: 199 CALORIES (3% FROM FAT)
FAT 0.6G (SATURATED FAT 0.1G)
PROTEIN 1.2G CARBOHYDRATE 50.4G
CHOLESTEROL 0MG SODIUM 10MG

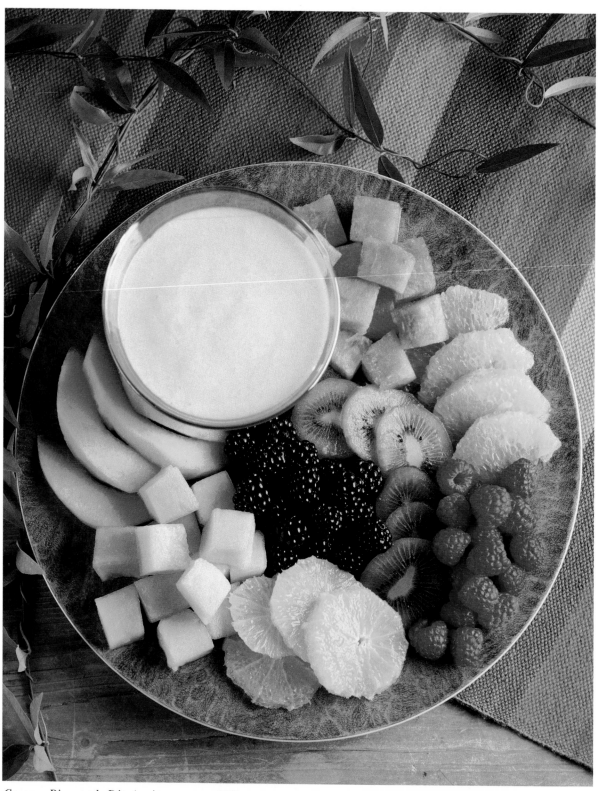

Creamy Pineapple Dip (recipe on page 122)

SNACKS & DESSERTS

*T*he best way to lose weight is to eat as little as possible, right? Wrong! The best way to lose weight and keep it off is to eat a variety of healthy foods that are low in calories and high in nutrients. And that includes snacks and desserts.

Using fruits, vegetables, breads, and low-fat dairy products, you can prepare low-calorie snacks with little fat. For instance, enjoy Orange-Pineapple Slush (page 121) or Crispy Snack Mix (page 124). And be sure to try Apricot Scones (page 130) with a cup of tea—delicious!

For a cool, healthy dessert, try Fresh Fruit with Strawberry Sauce (page 132) or one of the frozen yogurts on page 134.

SPICY TOMATO SIPPER

2¾ cups no-salt-added tomato juice
2 tablespoons lime juice
2 teaspoons low-sodium Worcestershire sauce
1 teaspoon prepared horseradish
½ teaspoon celery salt
¼ teaspoon hot sauce
Lime curls (optional)

Combine first 6 ingredients in a small pitcher; stir well. Cover and chill thoroughly. Garnish with lime curls, if desired. Yield: 3 (1-cup) servings.

PER SERVING: 51 CALORIES (0% FROM FAT)
FAT 0.0G (SATURATED FAT 0.0G)
PROTEIN 2.3G CARBOHYDRATE 12.9G
CHOLESTEROL 0MG SODIUM 390MG

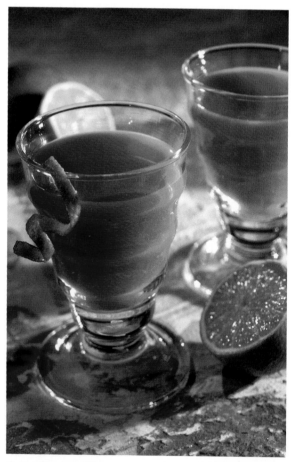

Spicy Tomato Sipper

ZIPPY RED-EYE

Increase tomato juice to 3¼ cups and hot sauce to ½ teaspoon. Continue with recipe as directed. Just before serving, stir in ½ cup vodka. Serve over ice. Garnish with celery sticks, if desired. Yield: 4 (1-cup) servings.

PER SERVING: 110 CALORIES (0% FROM FAT)
FAT 0.0G (SATURATED FAT 0.0G)
PROTEIN 2.0G CARBOHYDRATE 11.2G
CHOLESTEROL 0MG SODIUM 298MG

SPICED ORANGE CIDER

1 teaspoon grated orange rind
¼ teaspoon ground cinnamon
⅛ teaspoon ground allspice
2 whole cloves
1¾ cups unsweetened apple cider
½ cup unsweetened orange juice
2 (3-inch) sticks cinnamon (optional)

Place first 4 ingredients on a 4-inch square of cheesecloth or coffee filter; tie with string.
Pour cider and orange juice into a small saucepan; add spice bag. Cook over low heat 15 minutes, stirring occasionally. Remove and discard spice bag. Pour cider into mugs. Garnish with cinnamon sticks, if desired. Yield: 2 (1-cup) servings.

PER SERVING: 123 CALORIES (1% FROM FAT)
FAT 0.2G (SATURATED FAT 0.0G)
PROTEIN 0.5G CARBOHYDRATE 30.3G
CHOLESTEROL 0MG SODIUM 7MG

Calorie Tip-Off

When the food label says fat-free, it doesn't necessarily mean calorie-free. Manufacturers may use large amounts of carbohydrates and sugar to replace fat in products. And extra sugar can mean extra calories.
So instead of eating two fat-free muffins, eat one and keep fat and calories under control.

VIENNESE COFFEE

If you're a fan of flavored coffees, try this recipe using hazelnut, French vanilla, or cinnamon-flavored coffee. It's also delicious made with decaffeinated coffee.

1½ cups strong brewed coffee
½ cup skim milk
1 tablespoon sugar
1 teaspoon brandy extract
¼ cup frozen reduced-calorie whipped topping, thawed
Ground nutmeg (optional)

Combine first 4 ingredients in a small saucepan; cook over medium heat until thoroughly heated, stirring occasionally. Pour mixture evenly into 2 serving mugs; top each serving with 2 tablespoons whipped topping. Garnish with nutmeg, if desired. Serve immediately. Yield: 2 (1-cup) servings.

PER SERVING: 77 CALORIES (14% FROM FAT)
FAT 1.2G (SATURATED FAT 0.8G)
PROTEIN 2.5G CARBOHYDRATE 11.8G
CHOLESTEROL 1MG SODIUM 41MG

TROPICAL FRUIT SMOOTHIE

½ pound soft tofu, drained
1 cup sliced banana (about 1 medium)
2 cups unsweetened orange-pineapple juice, chilled
1 (8-ounce) can unsweetened crushed pineapple, undrained and chilled

Combine all ingredients in container of an electric blender; cover and process until smooth. Serve immediately. Yield: 5 (1-cup) servings.

PER SERVING: 133 CALORIES (10% FROM FAT)
FAT 1.5G (SATURATED FAT 0.2G)
PROTEIN 3.5G CARBOHYDRATE 28.4G
CHOLESTEROL 0MG SODIUM 3MG

RASPBERRY-BANANA FROSTY

1 cup frozen unsweetened raspberries
½ cup peeled, sliced banana
½ cup crushed ice
¼ cup skim milk
1 tablespoon sugar

Combine all ingredients in container of an electric blender; cover and process until smooth. Serve immediately. Yield: 3 (½-cup) servings.

PER SERVING: 66 CALORIES (5% FROM FAT)
FAT 0.4G (SATURATED FAT 0.1G)
PROTEIN 1.3G CARBOHYDRATE 15.7G
CHOLESTEROL 0MG SODIUM 11MG

WATERMELON SLUSH

8 cups cubed seeded watermelon
¼ cup sifted powdered sugar
1 (6-ounce) can frozen lemonade concentrate, thawed and undiluted
Mint sprigs (optional)

Place watermelon in a large bowl; cover and freeze.
Place half of frozen watermelon, half of powdered sugar, and half of concentrate in container of an electric blender; cover and process until smooth. Pour mixture into individual glasses.
Repeat procedure with remaining watermelon, powdered sugar, and concentrate. Garnish with mint sprigs, if desired. Serve immediately. Yield: 7 (1-cup) servings.

PER SERVING: 119 CALORIES (6% FROM FAT)
FAT 0.8G (SATURATED FAT 0.4G)
PROTEIN 1.2G CARBOHYDRATE 28.8G
CHOLESTEROL 0MG SODIUM 5MG

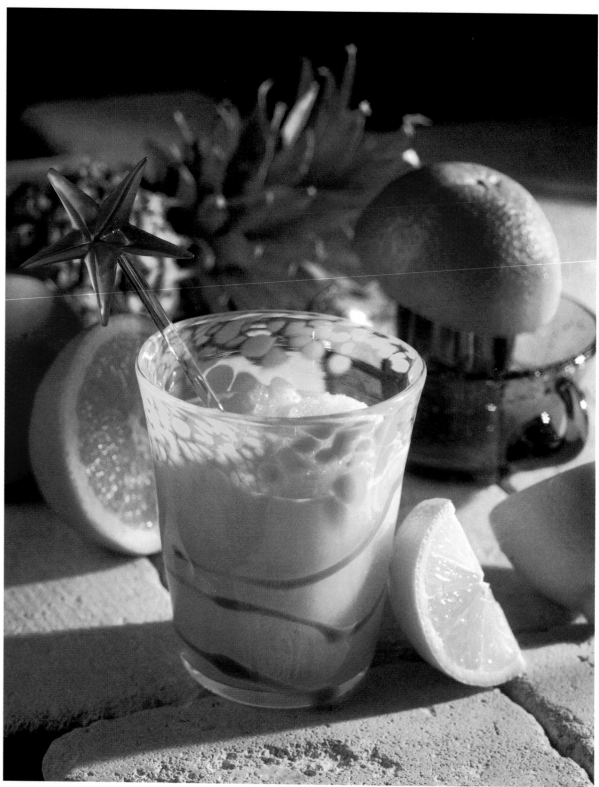

Orange-Pineapple Slush

ORANGE-PINEAPPLE SLUSH

3 cups ice cubes
1 cup freshly squeezed orange juice
½ cup unsweetened pineapple juice
¼ cup freshly squeezed lemon juice
3 tablespoons sugar

Combine all ingredients in container of an electric blender or food processor; cover and process on high speed until smooth and frothy. Serve immediately. Yield: 4 (1-cup) servings.

PER SERVING: 86 CALORIES (1% FROM FAT)
FAT 0.1G (SATURATED FAT 0.1G)
PROTEIN 0.6G   CARBOHYDRATE 21.7G
CHOLESTEROL 0MG   SODIUM 1MG

VERY BERRY SLUSH

Substitute cranberry juice cocktail for orange juice; omit pineapple juice. Add 1 tablespoon raspberry lemonade concentrate, thawed, and ½ cup water. Continue with recipe as directed. Yield: 4 (1-cup) servings.

PER SERVING: 86 CALORIES (0% FROM FAT)
FAT 0.0G (SATURATED FAT 0.0G)
PROTEIN 0.1G   CARBOHYDRATE 22.5G
CHOLESTEROL 0MG   SODIUM 3MG

FRUIT-YOGURT SWIRL

½ cup drained canned unsweetened pineapple
   chunks, chilled
½ cup drained canned unsweetened sliced
   peaches, chilled
5 ice cubes
3 whole fresh strawberries, caps removed
1 medium-size ripe banana, frozen
1 (8-ounce) carton low-fat vanilla yogurt

Combine all ingredients in container of an electric blender; cover and process until smooth. Pour into glasses, and serve immediately. Yield: 3 (1-cup) servings.

PER SERVING: 141 CALORIES (8% FROM FAT)
FAT 1.2G (SATURATED FAT 0.7G)
PROTEIN 4.4G   CARBOHYDRATE 29.7G
CHOLESTEROL 4MG   SODIUM 51MG

PEACH FRAPPÉ

1¼ cups frozen unsweetened sliced peaches
½ cup plain nonfat yogurt
½ cup unsweetened orange juice
2 teaspoons sugar

Combine all ingredients in container of an electric blender; cover and process until smooth. Serve immediately. Yield: 4 (½-cup) servings.

PER SERVING: 61 CALORIES (2% FROM FAT)
FAT 0.1G (SATURATED FAT 0.0G)
PROTEIN 2.2G   CARBOHYDRATE 13.5G
CHOLESTEROL 1MG   SODIUM 22MG

Focus on Fitness

If you're overweight or have a medical problem that forces you to limit high-impact sports, you may find water workouts to be your answer to achieving total fitness.

Water aerobics provides an excellent workout for the heart and muscles, and it burns lots of calories. The risk of injury is less than that from regular aerobics because the water acts as a cushion. Be sure to check with your physician before starting this or any other fitness program.

FRUIT SALSA WITH GRANOLA TOPPING

If covered tightly, this fruit mixture will keep in the refrigerator up to three days.

3 medium plums, pitted and diced
2 medium navel oranges, peeled, sectioned, and chopped
1 medium peach, pitted and diced
1 cup fresh raspberries
1 tablespoon minced fresh mint
1 tablespoon minced crystallized ginger
1 tablespoon fresh lime juice
2 teaspoons sugar
1 teaspoon grated orange rind
⅔ cup fresh orange juice
1 cup low-fat granola without raisins

Combine first 10 ingredients in a large bowl; toss gently. Cover and chill. To serve, spoon ½ cup fruit mixture into each individual serving bowl; top each with 2 tablespoons granola. Yield: 8 servings.

PER SERVING: 116 CALORIES (9% FROM FAT)
FAT 1.2G (SATURATED FAT 0.0G)
PROTEIN 2.0G   CARBOHYDRATE 27.2G
CHOLESTEROL 0MG   SODIUM 14MG

CINNAMON TORTILLA CHIPS WITH COFFEE DIP

6 (6-inch) flour tortillas
Vegetable cooking spray
2 tablespoons sugar
1 teaspoon unsweetened cocoa
¼ teaspoon ground cinnamon
1 cup frozen reduced-calorie whipped topping, thawed
½ cup coffee-flavored low-fat yogurt

Cut each tortilla into 6 wedges, and arrange in a single layer on a large baking sheet coated with cooking spray. Combine sugar, cocoa, and cinnamon, stirring well. Coat wedges with cooking spray; sprinkle half of sugar mixture over wedges. Turn wedges, and coat again with cooking spray; sprinkle remaining sugar mixture over wedges. Bake at 350° for 15 minutes or until crisp.
Combine whipped topping and yogurt, stirring well. Arrange 3 tortilla wedges around 2 tablespoons dip for each serving. Yield: 12 servings.

PER SERVING: 76 CALORIES (24% FROM FAT)
FAT 2.0G (SATURATED FAT 0.7G)
PROTEIN 1.9G   CARBOHYDRATE 12.7G
CHOLESTEROL 1MG   SODIUM 78MG

CREAMY PINEAPPLE DIP

(pictured on page 116)

1 cup lemon low-fat yogurt
3 tablespoons frozen pineapple juice concentrate, thawed and undiluted
1 tablespoon nonfat sour cream

Combine all ingredients in a bowl; stir well. Cover and chill at least 25 minutes. Stir before serving. Serve with fresh fruit. Store dip, tightly covered, in refrigerator up to 5 days. Yield: 1¼ cups.

PER TABLESPOON: 22 CALORIES (4% FROM FAT)
FAT 0.1G (SATURATED FAT 0.1G)
PROTEIN 0.5G   CARBOHYDRATE 4.7G
CHOLESTEROL 0MG   SODIUM 9MG

FYI

Food companies and health food stores often promote fruit juice sweeteners or honey as a healthier alternative to refined, or white, sugar. But using fruit sugar or honey to sweeten cookies or cakes offers no real nutritional advantage. Sugar is sugar, no matter what the source.
The only way fruit sugar has an advantage over other sugars is when it is still in the fruit. Then you get the fiber and other nutrients along with the sweetness!

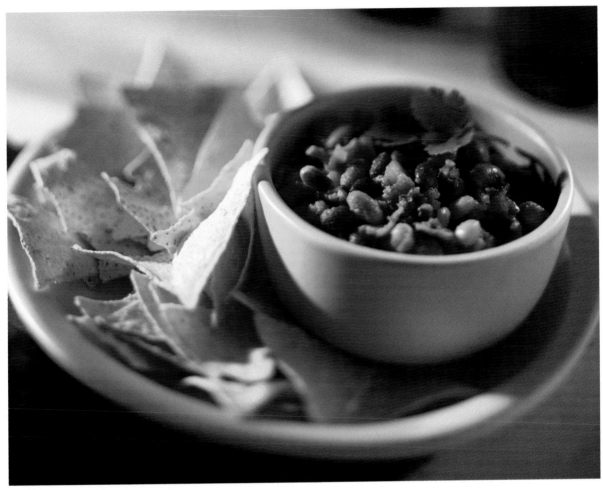

Buckaroo Bean and Bacon Salsa

BUCKAROO BEAN AND BACON SALSA

Vegetable cooking spray
1 cup chopped onion
2 cloves garlic, minced
1 (15-ounce) can black-eyed peas, rinsed and
    drained
1 (15-ounce) can black beans, rinsed and
    drained
1 (15-ounce) can pinquito or pinto beans,
    rinsed and drained
1 (14.5-ounce) can salsa with chipotle
1 (14.5-ounce) can salsa with cilantro
4 bacon slices, cooked, drained, and crumbled
2 tablespoons chopped fresh cilantro
Fresh cilantro sprigs (optional)

Coat a large nonstick skillet with cooking spray; place over medium heat. Add onion; sauté 5 minutes or until tender. Add garlic; sauté 1 minute. Add peas, beans, salsas, and bacon; cover and cook until thoroughly heated. Remove from heat; stir in chopped cilantro. Garnish with cilantro sprigs, if desired. Serve salsa warm with fat-free tortilla chips. Yield: 7 (½-cup) servings.

PER SERVING: 91 CALORIES (7% FROM FAT)
FAT 0.7G (SATURATED FAT 0.2G)
PROTEIN 5.4G   CARBOHYDRATE 17.1G
CHOLESTEROL 1MG   SODIUM 301MG

PEPPERED CHEESE CHIPS

3 (6-inch) flour tortillas
Vegetable cooking spray
1 tablespoon grated Parmesan cheese
⅛ teaspoon ground red pepper
⅛ teaspoon black pepper

Coat tortillas with cooking spray; cut each into 4 wedges. Combine cheese and peppers. Stir well; sprinkle over wedges. Arrange on a baking sheet. Bake at 350° for 10 minutes. Yield: 1 dozen chips.

PER CHIP: 28 CALORIES (26% FROM FAT)
FAT 0.8G (SATURATED FAT 0.2G)
PROTEIN 0.8G   CARBOHYDRATE 4.2G
CHOLESTEROL 0MG   SODIUM 44MG

CRISPY SNACK MIX

(pictured on page 131)

1½ cups small unsalted pretzels
1 cup bite-size shredded whole wheat cereal biscuits
1 cup bite-size corn-and-rice cereal
1 cup commercial plain croutons
¾ cup bite-size crispy bran squares
2 tablespoons reduced-calorie margarine
1 tablespoon low-sodium Worcestershire sauce
2 teaspoons dried Italian seasoning
¼ teaspoon pepper
⅛ teaspoon salt
⅛ teaspoon garlic powder
2 tablespoons grated Parmesan cheese

Combine first 5 ingredients. Toss and set aside.
Combine margarine and next 5 ingredients in a saucepan; cook over medium heat, stirring frequently, until margarine melts. Pour over cereal mixture. Sprinkle with cheese; toss well.
Spread mixture in a 13- x 9- x 2-inch baking dish. Bake at 275° for 45 minutes or until crisp, stirring occasionally. Cool. Yield: 10 (½-cup) servings.

PER SERVING: 103 CALORIES (24% FROM FAT)
FAT 2.7G (SATURATED FAT 0.4G)
PROTEIN 2.7G   CARBOHYDRATE 18.0G
CHOLESTEROL 1MG   SODIUM 219MG

GROUND BEEF AND CHEESE SNACKS

Vegetable cooking spray
½ pound ground round
⅔ cup chopped green pepper
½ cup chopped onion
1 clove garlic, minced
¾ cup (3 ounces) shredded reduced-fat sharp Cheddar cheese
¾ cup (3 ounces) shredded part-skim mozzarella cheese
⅓ cup no-salt-added tomato sauce
¾ teaspoon dried Italian seasoning
¼ teaspoon freshly ground pepper
1 (11-ounce) package refrigerated crusty French loaf dough
1 tablespoon grated Parmesan cheese

Coat a large nonstick skillet with cooking spray; add ground round and next 3 ingredients. Cook over medium heat until meat is browned, stirring until it crumbles. Drain and pat dry with paper towels. Wipe drippings from skillet with a paper towel.
Combine meat mixture, Cheddar cheese, and next 4 ingredients; stir well.
Unroll dough into a large rectangle; cut into 36 (2-inch) squares. Place squares on a large baking sheet coated with cooking spray. Spoon about 1½ teaspoons meat mixture onto each dough square. Sprinkle Parmesan cheese evenly over squares.
Bake at 425° for 10 to 12 minutes or until crust is crisp and lightly browned. Serve warm. Yield: 3 dozen snacks.
Note: Meat mixture may be prepared ahead. Combine cooked meat mixture, Cheddar cheese, and next 4 ingredients; place in an airtight container. Refrigerate up to 24 hours. Remove meat mixture from refrigerator; assemble and cook appetizers as directed above.

PER SNACK: 50 CALORIES (29% FROM FAT)
FAT 1.6G (SATURATED FAT 0.7G)
PROTEIN 3.9G   CARBOHYDRATE 4.7G
CHOLESTEROL 8MG   SODIUM 79MG

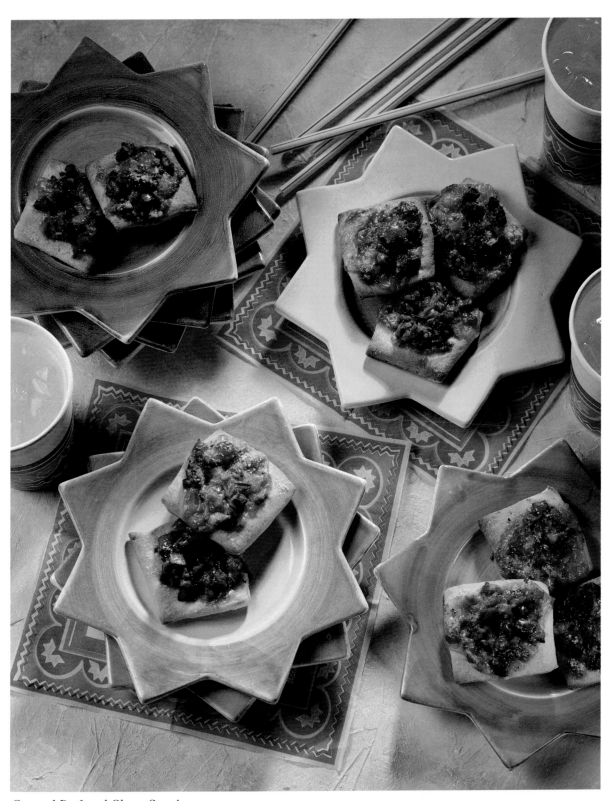

Ground Beef and Cheese Snacks

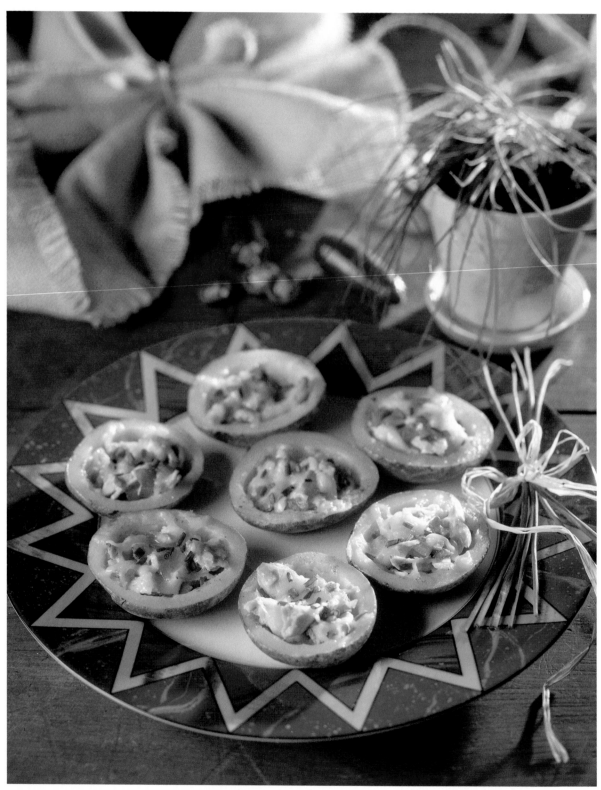

Chicken-Chile Potato Skins

HAM BITES

3 ounces Neufchâtel cheese, softened
½ cup shredded baking apple
2 tablespoons chopped onion
2 teaspoons Dijon mustard
1 cup finely chopped reduced-fat, low-salt ham
12 miniature bagels, split
¼ cup (1 ounce) finely shredded smoked
   Gouda cheese

Combine first 4 ingredients. Stir in ham. Spread ham mixture evenly over bagel halves. Place on an ungreased baking sheet, and bake at 375° for 10 minutes. Sprinkle bagels with Gouda cheese, and bake 5 minutes or until cheese melts. Yield: 2 dozen snacks.

PER SNACK: 59 CALORIES (26% FROM FAT)
FAT 1.7G (SATURATED FAT 0.9G)
PROTEIN 3.1G CARBOHYDRATE 7.7G
CHOLESTEROL 7MG SODIUM 150MG

CHICKEN-CHILE POTATO SKINS

8 (5-ounce) baking potatoes
Butter-flavored vegetable cooking spray
¼ teaspoon garlic powder
¼ teaspoon salt
¼ teaspoon ground red pepper
1 cup shredded cooked chicken
3 tablespoons chopped green chiles
1 small jalapeño pepper, seeded and minced
1 cup (4 ounces) shredded reduced-fat
   Monterey Jack cheese
Chopped fresh chives (optional)

Wash potatoes; pat dry. Prick each potato several times with a fork. Arrange 4 potatoes in a circle 1 inch apart on a layer of paper towels in microwave oven. Microwave, uncovered, at HIGH 8 to 10 minutes or until potatoes are tender, turning and rearranging potatoes halfway through cooking time. Repeat procedure with remaining 4 potatoes. Let potatoes cool to touch.

Cut each potato in half lengthwise; scoop out pulp, leaving ¼-inch-thick shells. Reserve pulp for another use. Place potato shells on an ungreased baking sheet. Spray shells with cooking spray.
Combine garlic powder, salt, and red pepper; sprinkle evenly over shells.
Combine chicken, chiles, and jalapeño pepper; spoon evenly into shells.
Sprinkle with cheese. Bake at 450° for 4 to 6 minutes or until cheese melts. Garnish with chives, if desired. Yield: 16 snacks.

PER SNACK: 82 CALORIES (23% FROM FAT)
FAT 2.1G (SATURATED FAT 1.0G)
PROTEIN 4.9G CARBOHYDRATE 11.1G
CHOLESTEROL 10MG SODIUM 98MG

VEGGIE QUESADILLAS

Butter-flavored vegetable cooking spray
½ cup finely shredded cabbage
¼ cup finely chopped fresh mushrooms
2 tablespoons finely chopped sweet red pepper
2 tablespoons finely shredded carrot
1 tablespoon minced onion
⅛ teaspoon ground celery seeds
Dash of salt
2 (6-inch) flour tortillas
¼ cup (1 ounce) shredded reduced-fat sharp
   Cheddar cheese

Coat a small nonstick skillet with cooking spray; place over medium-high heat until hot. Add cabbage and next 6 ingredients; sauté 5 minutes or until vegetables are tender.
Spoon vegetable mixture over 1 tortilla; spread to within ½ inch of edge. Sprinkle with cheese, and top with remaining tortilla.
Coat skillet with cooking spray, and place over medium-high heat until hot. Add quesadilla, and cook 2 minutes on each side or until lightly browned. Remove from skillet; cut into 4 wedges, and serve immediately. Yield: 4 snacks.

PER SNACK: 89 CALORIES (30% FROM FAT)
FAT 3.0G (SATURATED FAT 1.0G)
PROTEIN 3.9G CARBOHYDRATE 11.6G
CHOLESTEROL 5MG SODIUM 173MG

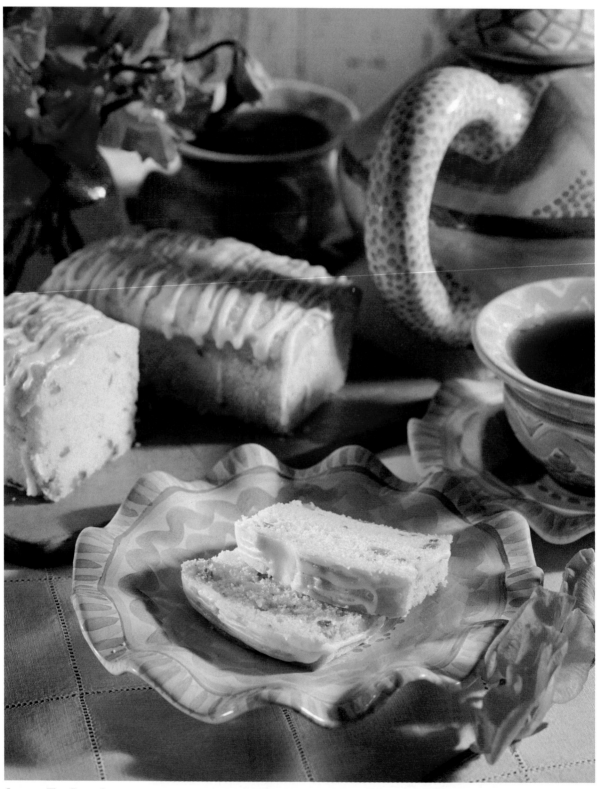

Lemon Tea Bread

LEMON TEA BREAD

You may substitute 1 teaspoon lemon extract for the lemon rind, if desired.

¼ cup margarine, softened
½ (8-ounce) package nonfat cream cheese, softened
⅔ cup sugar
1 egg
2 teaspoons grated lemon rind
1 cup all-purpose flour
1½ teaspoons baking powder
¼ teaspoon salt
½ cup skim milk
¼ cup chopped pecans
Vegetable cooking spray
⅓ cup sifted powdered sugar
2 teaspoons lemon juice

Beat margarine and cream cheese at medium speed of an electric mixer until creamy; gradually add ⅔ cup sugar, beating well. Add egg and lemon rind, beating just until blended.

Combine flour, baking powder, and salt; add to margarine mixture alternately with milk, beginning and ending with flour mixture. Mix at low speed after each addition until blended. Stir in pecans.

Pour batter into 2 (5¾- x 3¼- x 2-inch) loafpans coated with cooking spray. Bake at 325° for 40 to 45 minutes or until a wooden pick inserted in center comes out clean. Cool bread in pans on wire racks 5 minutes; remove from pans, and let cool slightly.

Combine powdered sugar and lemon juice in a small bowl, stirring until blended. Drizzle glaze over tops of loaves. Serve warm or at room temperature. To serve, cut each loaf into 8 slices. Yield: 16 slices.

PER SLICE: 122 CALORIES (33% FROM FAT)
FAT 4.5G (SATURATED FAT 0.8G)
PROTEIN 2.7G   CARBOHYDRATE 18.0G
CHOLESTEROL 15MG   SODIUM 121MG

LEMON-CURRANT BREAD

Fold ¼ cup currants into Lemon Tea Bread batter with the pecans. Bake as directed.

PER SLICE: 129 CALORIES (32% FROM FAT)
FAT 4.6G (SATURATED FAT 0.8G)
PROTEIN 2.7G   CARBOHYDRATE 19.5G
CHOLESTEROL 15MG   SODIUM 122MG

BANANA YOGURT BREAD

2 cups all-purpose flour
1½ teaspoons baking powder
½ teaspoon baking soda
½ teaspoon salt
1 (8-ounce) carton plain nonfat yogurt
1 cup mashed ripe banana
½ cup sugar
¼ cup margarine, melted
1 teaspoon vanilla extract
2 egg whites, lightly beaten
1 egg, lightly beaten
Vegetable cooking spray
2 teaspoons all-purpose flour

Combine first 4 ingredients in a large bowl; make a well in center of mixture. Combine yogurt and next 6 ingredients; add to dry ingredients, stirring just until dry ingredients are moistened.

Coat a 9- x 5- x 3-inch loafpan with cooking spray; sprinkle with 2 teaspoons flour. Spoon batter into prepared pan. Bake at 350° for 1 hour or until a wooden pick inserted in center comes out clean. Let cool in pan 10 minutes; remove from pan, and let cool on a wire rack. Yield: 18 (½-inch) slices.

PER SLICE: 123 CALORIES (22% FROM FAT)
FAT 3.1G (SATURATED FAT 0.7G)
PROTEIN 3.1G   CARBOHYDRATE 20.9G
CHOLESTEROL 13MG   SODIUM 162MG

APRICOT SCONES

2 cups all-purpose flour
1½ teaspoons baking powder
½ teaspoon baking soda
¼ teaspoon salt
¼ cup sugar
¼ cup margarine, chilled and cut into pieces
⅓ cup chopped dried apricots
¼ cup nonfat buttermilk
¼ cup apricot nectar
1 egg, lightly beaten
Vegetable cooking spray
1 egg white, lightly beaten
1 tablespoon sugar

Combine first 5 ingredients in a bowl; cut in margarine with a pastry blender until mixture resembles coarse meal. Add apricots; toss well. Combine buttermilk, nectar, and egg; add to dry ingredients, stirring just until moistened. (Dough will be sticky.)

Turn out onto a lightly floured surface; knead 4 to 5 times. Pat into a 9-inch circle on a baking sheet coated with cooking spray. Cut into 12 wedges, cutting to, but not through, bottom of dough. Brush with egg white; sprinkle with 1 tablespoon sugar. Bake at 400° for 15 minutes. Yield: 1 dozen.

PER SCONE: 149 CALORIES (27% FROM FAT)
FAT 4.5G (SATURATED FAT 0.9G)
PROTEIN 3.2G CARBOHYDRATE 24.0G
CHOLESTEROL 18MG SODIUM 184MG

ALMOND BISCOTTI

2 eggs
1 egg white
¼ cup sugar
¼ teaspoon almond extract
2⅓ cups all-purpose flour
¾ teaspoon baking soda
¼ teaspoon salt
½ cup sugar
¼ cup chocolate wafer crumbs
1 (2-ounce) package slivered almonds,
    coarsely chopped and toasted
Vegetable cooking spray

Beat eggs and egg white at high speed of an electric mixer 3 minutes. Gradually add ¼ cup sugar, beating at high speed. Add almond extract, and beat 2 additional minutes.

Combine flour and next 4 ingredients in a medium bowl, stirring well; stir in almonds. Slowly add egg mixture to flour mixture, stirring until dry ingredients are moistened. (Mixture will be stiff.)

Turn dough out onto lightly floured surface, and knead lightly 7 or 8 times. Divide dough in half; shape each half into an 8-inch log. Place logs, 4 inches apart, on a baking sheet coated with cooking spray. Bake at 350° for 40 minutes. Remove from oven, and let cool 15 minutes.

Using a serrated knife, cut each log diagonally into 15 (½-inch-thick) slices; place slices, cut side down, on baking sheet. Reduce oven temperature to 300°, and bake 23 minutes. (Cookies will be slightly soft in center but will harden as they cool.) Remove from baking sheet, and let cool completely on wire racks. Yield: 2½ dozen.

PER COOKIE: 75 CALORIES (19% FROM FAT)
FAT 1.6G (SATURATED FAT 0.3G)
PROTEIN 2.0G CARBOHYDRATE 13.3G
CHOLESTEROL 15MG SODIUM 60MG

LAYERED FRUIT POPS

If fresh peaches are not available, you may use frozen unsweetened peaches instead.

1½ cups fresh orange juice
¼ cup sugar
¼ cup plus 2 tablespoons fresh lemon juice
¼ teaspoon ground cinnamon
4 cups fresh strawberries, sliced
4 cups chopped fresh peaches
14 (6-ounce) paper cups
14 wooden sticks

Combine first 4 ingredients in container of an electric blender; cover and process until combined, stopping once to scrape down sides. Reserve 1 cup orange juice mixture; set aside. Add strawberries to remaining juice in blender; process until smooth. Transfer strawberry mixture to a bowl; set aside.

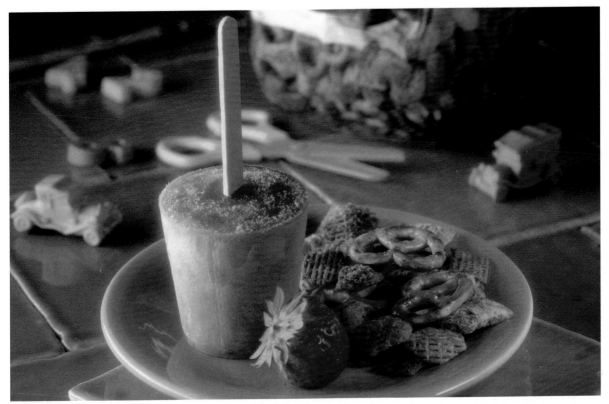

Strawberry Yogurt Pops and Crispy Snack Mix (page 124)

Combine reserved 1 cup orange juice mixture and peaches in blender; cover and process until smooth. Transfer mixture to a bowl.

Spoon 2 tablespoons strawberry mixture into each paper cup. Cover tops of cups with aluminum foil, and insert a wooden stick through foil into center of each cup. Freeze until firm.

Pour 2 tablespoons peach mixture over frozen strawberry mixture in each cup. Freeze until firm. Repeat procedure with remaining strawberry and peach mixtures. To serve, remove aluminum foil; peel cup from pop. Yield: 14 pops.

PER POP: 56 CALORIES (3% FROM FAT)
FAT 0.2G (SATURATED FAT 0.0G)
PROTEIN 0.7G   CARBOHYDRATE 14.1G
CHOLESTEROL 0MG   SODIUM 1MG

STRAWBERRY YOGURT POPS

1 (16-ounce) package frozen unsweetened
    strawberries, thawed and crushed
1 (8-ounce) carton strawberry low-fat yogurt
⅔ cup cranberry juice cocktail
1 tablespoon sugar
10 (3-ounce) paper cups
10 wooden sticks

Combine first 4 ingredients in a medium bowl, stirring well. Spoon mixture evenly into paper cups. Insert a wooden stick into center of each cup, and freeze until firm. To serve, peel cup from pop. Yield: 10 pops.

PER POP: 53 CALORIES (5% FROM FAT)
FAT 0.3G (SATURATED FAT 0.2G)
PROTEIN 1.1G   CARBOHYDRATE 12.2G
CHOLESTEROL 1MG   SODIUM 14MG

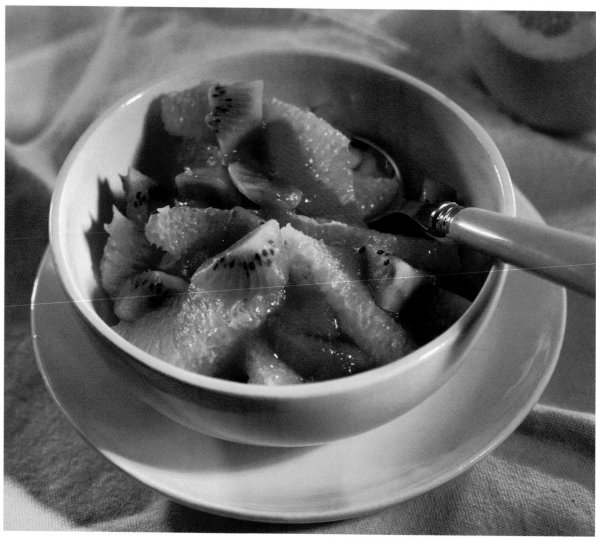

Fresh Fruit with Strawberry Sauce

FRESH FRUIT WITH STRAWBERRY SAUCE

Serve this fresh-tasting sauce over nonfat frozen yogurt, ice cream, or angel food cake.

1 cup frozen unsweetened whole strawberries, thawed
2 teaspoons sugar
¼ teaspoon grated orange rind
2 cups orange sections (about 6 oranges)
1 cup cubed peeled kiwifruit (about 3 kiwifruit)

Place first 3 ingredients in container of an electric blender; cover and process until smooth. Set aside.

Spoon ½ cup orange sections and ¼ cup kiwifruit into each of 4 small bowls; top each serving with 3 tablespoons sauce. Yield: 4 servings.

PER SERVING: 99 CALORIES (5% FROM FAT)
FAT 0.5G (SATURATED FAT 0.1G)
PROTEIN 1.8G CARBOHYDRATE 23.3G
CHOLESTEROL 0MG SODIUM 1MG

CRANBERRY-PINEAPPLE ICE

4½ cups water, divided
2¼ cups fresh cranberries
1¼ cups sugar, divided
1 cup unsweetened pineapple juice
3 tablespoons unsweetened orange juice
Fresh mint sprigs (optional)

Combine ¾ cup water, cranberries, and ½ cup sugar in a small saucepan; stir well. Bring cranberry mixture to a boil over medium heat; cook 8 minutes or until cranberries pop, stirring frequently. Remove from heat, and let cool.

Position knife blade in food processor bowl. Add cranberry mixture; process until smooth. Strain puree through a sieve; discard pulp.

Combine cranberry puree, remaining 3¾ cups water, remaining ¾ cup sugar, pineapple juice, and orange juice in a large bowl; stir well.

Pour cranberry mixture into freezer can of a 1-gallon hand-turned or electric freezer. Freeze according to manufacturer's instructions. Pack freezer with additional ice and rock salt; let stand 1 hour, if desired.

Scoop mixture into individual dessert bowls. Garnish with mint sprigs, if desired. Serve immediately. Yield: 20 (½-cup) servings.

PER SERVING: 63 CALORIES (0% FROM FAT)
FAT 0.0G (SATURATED FAT 0.0G)
PROTEIN 0.1G CARBOHYDRATE 16.1G
CHOLESTEROL 0MG SODIUM 0MG

BERRY ICE MILK

⅔ cup fresh raspberries
⅔ cup sugar
2 cups sliced fresh strawberries
2 teaspoons lemon juice
1 cup evaporated skimmed milk
1 (4-ounce) carton frozen egg substitute, thawed
1 cup 2% low-fat milk

Place raspberries in food processor, and process until smooth. Press puree through a sieve; set puree aside, and discard seeds.

Combine sugar, strawberries, and lemon juice in processor, and process until smooth. Add raspberry puree, evaporated milk, and egg substitute, and process until blended. Pour mixture into a large bowl, and stir in low-fat milk.

Pour berry mixture into freezer can of a 2-quart hand-turned or electric freezer, and freeze according to manufacturer's instructions. Spoon into a freezer-safe container; cover and freeze for at least 1 hour. Yield: 14 (½-cup) servings.

PER SERVING: 73 CALORIES (6% FROM FAT)
FAT 0.5G (SATURATED 0.2G)
PROTEIN 3.0G CARBOHYDRATE 14.8G
CHOLESTEROL 2MG SODIUM 42MG

REFRESHING CITRUS SORBET

3½ cups water
½ cup sugar
1 (6-ounce) can frozen orange juice concentrate, undiluted
1 tablespoon grated lime rind
1 tablespoon grated lemon rind
1 tablespoon fresh lime juice
1 tablespoon fresh lemon juice

Combine water and sugar in a saucepan; stir well. Bring to a boil; reduce heat, and simmer, stirring until sugar dissolves. Let cool to room temperature.

Combine sugar mixture, orange juice concentrate, and remaining ingredients in container of an electric blender; cover and process until smooth.

Pour mixture into freezer can of a 2-quart hand-turned or electric freezer. Freeze according to manufacturer's instructions. Let ripen 1 hour, if desired. Scoop sorbet into individual dessert bowls. Serve immediately. Yield: 8 (½-cup) servings.

PER SERVING: 83 CALORIES (1% FROM FAT)
FAT 0.1G (SATURATED FAT 0.0G)
PROTEIN 0.5G CARBOHYDRATE 21.2G
CHOLESTEROL 0MG SODIUM 1MG

VANILLA FROZEN YOGURT

2 envelopes unflavored gelatin
2 cups skim milk
1 cup sugar
Dash of salt
5 cups vanilla low-fat yogurt
1 tablespoon plus 1 teaspoon vanilla extract

Sprinkle gelatin over milk in a saucepan; let stand 1 minute. Cook over low heat, stirring constantly, until gelatin dissolves. Remove from heat; add sugar and salt, stirring until sugar dissolves. Stir in yogurt and vanilla. Cover and chill 1 hour.

Pour yogurt mixture into freezer can of a 1-gallon hand-turned or electric freezer; freeze according to manufacturer's instructions. Scoop yogurt into individual bowls. Serve immediately. Yield: 22 (½-cup) servings.

PER SERVING: 92 CALORIES (7% FROM FAT)
FAT 0.7G (SATURATED FAT 0.4G)
PROTEIN 3.9G CARBOHYDRATE 17.5G
CHOLESTEROL 3MG SODIUM 53MG

STRAWBERRY FROZEN YOGURT

Add 6 cups fresh strawberries, hulled and pureed, to yogurt mixture before chilling. Proceed as directed above. Yield: 26 (½-cup) servings.

PER SERVING: 87 CALORIES (7% FROM FAT)
FAT 0.7G (SATURATED FAT 0.4G)
PROTEIN 3.4G CARBOHYDRATE 17.0G
CHOLESTEROL 3MG SODIUM 45MG

PEACH FROZEN YOGURT

Add 3 pounds fresh peaches, peeled, pitted, and pureed, to yogurt mixture before chilling. Pour into freezer can of a 5-quart hand-turned or electric freezer; freeze according to manufacturer's instructions. Yield: 30 (½-cup) servings.

PER SERVING: 80 CALORIES (6% FROM FAT)
FAT 0.5G (SATURATED FAT 0.3G)
PROTEIN 3.0G CARBOHYDRATE 16.2G
CHOLESTEROL 2MG SODIUM 39MG

RASPBERRY FROZEN YOGURT

½ cup skim milk
2 teaspoons cornstarch
½ cup light-colored corn syrup
1 (12-ounce) package frozen unsweetened raspberries, thawed
1 (8-ounce) carton vanilla low-fat yogurt
Crushed ice (optional)

Combine milk and cornstarch in a small saucepan; stir well. Cook over medium heat, stirring constantly, until mixture is thickened and bubbly. Remove from heat, and stir in corn syrup. Set milk mixture aside.

Place raspberries in container of an electric blender or food processor; cover and process 45 seconds or until smooth. Transfer to a wire-mesh strainer; press with back of spoon against sides of strainer to squeeze out juice. Discard seeds and pulp in strainer. Add raspberry juice and yogurt to milk mixture, stirring with a wire whisk until blended. Cover and chill thoroughly.

Pour mixture into freezer can of a 2-quart hand-turned or electric freezer, and freeze according to manufacturer's instructions. Pack freezer with additional ice and rock salt, and let stand 1 hour. Scoop into individual dessert bowls. Place bowls on crushed ice before serving, if desired. Serve immediately. Yield: 6 (½-cup) servings.

PER SERVING: 143 CALORIES (4% FROM FAT)
FAT 0.7G (SATURATED FAT 0.3G)
PROTEIN 2.9G CARBOHYDRATE 31.9G
CHOLESTEROL 2MG SODIUM 69MG

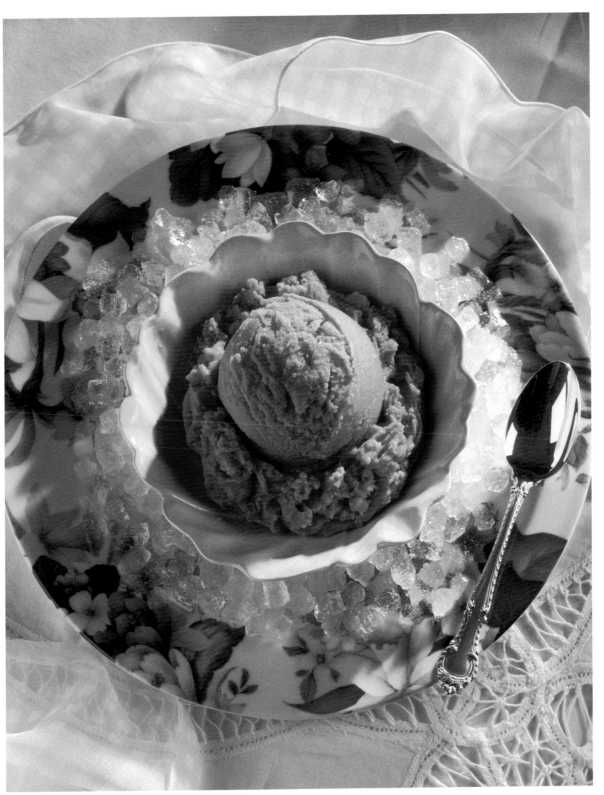

Raspberry Frozen Yogurt

CALORIE/NUTRIENT CHART

FOOD	APPROXIMATE MEASURE	FOOD ENERGY (CALORIES)	FAT (GRAMS)	SATURATED FAT (GRAMS)
Alfalfa sprouts	½ cup	8	0.2	0.02
Apple				
Fresh, with skin	1 medium	81	0.5	0.08
Juice, unsweetened	½ cup	58	0.1	0.02
Applesauce, unsweetened	½ cup	52	0.1	0.01
Apricot				
Fresh	1 each	18	0.1	0.01
Canned, in juice	½ cup	58	0.0	0.00
Nectar	½ cup	70	0.1	0.01
Artichoke				
Whole, cooked	1 each	53	0.2	0.04
Hearts, cooked	½ cup	37	0.1	0.03
Arugula	3 ounces	21	0.5	—
Asparagus, fresh, cooked, cut	½ cup	23	0.3	0.06
Avocado	1 medium	322	30.6	4.88
Bacon				
Canadian-style	1 ounce	45	2.0	0.63
Turkey, cooked	1 ounce	60	4.0	—
Bamboo shoots, cooked	½ cup	7	0.1	0.03
Banana	1 medium	109	0.5	0.22
Barley, cooked	½ cup	97	0.3	0.07
Bean sprouts, raw	½ cup	16	0.1	0.01
Beans, cooked and drained				
Black	½ cup	114	0.5	0.12
Cannellini or kidney	½ cup	112	0.4	0.06
Garbanzo (chickpeas)	½ cup	134	2.1	0.22
Green, fresh	½ cup	22	0.2	0.40
Lima, frozen, baby	½ cup	94	0.3	0.06
Pinto, canned, no-salt-added	½ cup	90	0.5	0.00
Beef, trimmed of fat				
Flank steak, broiled	3 ounces	207	12.7	5.43
Liver, braised	3 ounces	137	4.2	1.62
Round, top, lean, broiled	3 ounces	162	5.3	1.84
Sirloin, broiled	3 ounces	177	7.4	3.03
Tenderloin, roasted	3 ounces	173	7.9	3.09
Beets, fresh, diced, cooked	½ cup	26	0.4	0.01
Beverages				
Beer	12 fluid ounces	146	0.0	0.00
Beer, light	12 fluid ounces	95	0.0	0.00
Bourbon, brandy, rum, or whiskey, 80 proof	1 fluid ounce	65	0.0	0.00
Champagne	6 fluid ounces	135	0.0	0.00
Coffee, black	1 cup	5	0.0	0.00
Wine, red	6 fluid ounces	121	0.0	0.00
Wine, white, dry	6 fluid ounces	117	0.0	0.00
Biscuit and baking mix, low-fat	¼ cup	140	0.5	0.00
Blackberries, fresh	½ cup	37	0.3	0.01
Blueberries, fresh	½ cup	41	0.3	0.02
Bouillon, dry				
Beef-flavored granules	1 teaspoon	10	1.1	0.30
Chicken-flavored granules	1 teaspoon	10	1.1	0.30

FOOD	APPROXIMATE MEASURE	FOOD ENERGY (CALORIES)	FAT (GRAMS)	SATURATED FAT (GRAMS)
Bran				
Oat, dry, uncooked	½ cup	153	3.0	0.28
Oat, unprocessed	½ cup	114	3.3	0.62
Wheat, crude	½ cup	65	1.3	0.19
Bread				
Bagel, regular-size, plain	1 each	161	1.5	0.21
Biscuit, homemade	1 each	127	6.4	1.74
Bun, hamburger or hot dog	1 each	136	3.4	0.52
Bun, hamburger, reduced-calorie, whole wheat	1 each	80	1.0	0.00
Cornbread	2-ounce square	154	6.0	3.36
English muffin	1 each	182	3.6	1.93
French	1 slice	73	0.5	0.16
Light, Italian	1 slice	40	0.0	0.00
Pita, whole wheat	1 medium	122	0.9	0.10
Pumpernickel	1 slice	76	0.4	0.05
White	1 slice	67	0.8	0.19
Whole wheat	1 slice	56	0.7	0.12
Breadcrumbs				
Fine, dry	½ cup	196	2.2	0.52
Seasoned	½ cup	214	1.5	—
Breadstick, plain	1 each	17	0.5	—
Broccoli, fresh, chopped, cooked or raw	½ cup	12	0.1	0.02
Broth				
Beef, no-salt-added	1 cup	22	0.0	0.00
Chicken, no-salt-added	1 cup	16	1.0	—
Vegetable	1 cup	22	1.1	—
Brussels sprouts, fresh, cooked	½ cup	30	0.4	0.08
Bulgur, uncooked	½ cup	239	0.9	0.16
Butter	1 tablespoon	102	11.5	7.17
Cabbage, raw, shredded	½ cup	8	0.1	0.01
Cake, without frosting				
Angel food	2-ounce slice	147	0.1	—
Pound, fat-free	2-ounce slice	147	0.0	0.00
Yellow, cut into 12 slices	1 slice	190	7.5	1.92
Candy				
Caramels	1 ounce	108	2.3	1.87
Fudge, chocolate	1 ounce	113	3.4	—
Gumdrops	1 ounce	98	0.2	0.03
Jelly beans	1 ounce	104	0.1	0.09
Milk chocolate	1 ounce	153	8.7	5.13
Cantaloupe, raw, diced	½ cup	28	0.2	0.12
Capers	1 tablespoon	4	0.0	—
Carambola (starfruit)	1 medium	42	0.4	—
Carrot				
Raw	1 medium	31	0.1	0.02
Cooked, sliced	½ cup	33	0.1	0.22
Juice, canned	½ cup	66	0.2	0.05
Cauliflower, raw, flowerets	½ cup	12	0.1	0.01
Caviar	1 tablespoon	40	2.9	0.07

Dash (—) indicates insufficient data available.

FOOD	APPROXIMATE MEASURE	FOOD ENERGY (CALORIES)	FAT (GRAMS)	SATURATED FAT (GRAMS)
Celery, raw, diced	½ cup	10	0.1	0.02
Cereal				
Bran flakes	½ cup	64	0.4	0.06
Bran, whole	½ cup	104	1.5	0.12
Corn flakes	½ cup	44	0.0	0.00
Crispy rice	½ cup	55	0.1	—
Puffed wheat	½ cup	22	0.1	0.01
Raisin bran	½ cup	77	0.5	—
Shredded wheat miniatures	½ cup	76	0.5	0.08
Cheese				
American, light, process	1 ounce	50	2.0	—
Blue	1 ounce	100	8.1	5.30
Brie	1 ounce	95	7.8	4.94
Camembert	1 ounce	85	6.9	4.33
Cheddar, light, process	1 ounce	50	2.0	—
Cottage, nonfat	½ cup	70	0.0	0.00
Cottage, low-fat (1% milkfat)	½ cup	81	1.1	0.72
Cream, light	1 ounce	62	4.8	2.86
Cream, nonfat	1 ounce	24	0.0	—
Farmer	1 ounce	40	3.0	—
Feta	1 ounce	75	6.0	4.24
Fontina	1 ounce	110	8.8	5.44
Goat, semisoft	1 ounce	103	8.5	5.85
Gouda	1 ounce	101	7.8	4.99
Gruyère	1 ounce	117	9.2	5.36
Monterey Jack, reduced-fat	1 ounce	83	5.4	3.15
Mozzarella, part-skim	1 ounce	72	4.5	2.86
Neufchâtel	1 ounce	74	6.6	4.20
Parmesan, grated	1 ounce	129	8.5	5.40
Provolone	1 ounce	100	7.5	4.84
Ricotta, light	1 ounce	20	1.0	0.60
Ricotta, part-skim	1 ounce	39	2.2	1.39
Romano, grated	1 ounce	110	7.6	4.85
Swiss, reduced-fat	1 ounce	85	5.0	2.78
Cherries				
Fresh, sweet	½ cup	52	0.7	0.16
Sour, unsweetened	½ cup	39	0.2	0.05
Chicken, skinned, boned, and roasted				
White meat	3 ounces	147	3.8	1.07
Dark meat	3 ounces	174	8.3	2.26
Liver	3 ounces	134	4.6	1.56
Chili sauce	1 tablespoon	18	0.1	0.03
Chives, raw, chopped	1 tablespoon	1	0.0	0.00
Chocolate				
Chips, semisweet	¼ cup	215	15.2	—
Sweet	1 ounce	150	9.9	—
Unsweetened, baking	1 ounce	141	14.7	8.79
White, baking	1 ounce	169	11.9	7.18
Chutney, apple	1 tablespoon	41	0.0	—
Cilantro, fresh, minced	1 tablespoon	1	0.0	0.00
Clams, canned, drained	½ cup	118	1.6	0.15
Cocoa powder, unsweetened	1 tablespoon	24	0.7	0.44
Coconut				
Fresh, grated	1 cup	460	43.5	38.61
Dried, unsweetened, shredded	1 cup	526	51.4	45.62

FOOD	APPROXIMATE MEASURE	FOOD ENERGY (CALORIES)	FAT (GRAMS)	SATURATED FAT (GRAMS)
Cookies				
Brownie	2-ounce bar	243	10.1	3.13
Chocolate chip, homemade	1 each	69	4.6	—
Fortune	1 each	23	0.2	—
Gingersnaps	1 each	36	1.3	0.33
Vanilla creme	1 each	83	3.6	—
Vanilla wafers	1 each	17	0.9	0.17
Corn				
Fresh, kernels, cooked	½ cup	89	1.0	0.16
Cream-style, regular pack	½ cup	92	0.5	0.08
Cornmeal, degermed, yellow	1 cup	505	2.3	0.31
Cornstarch	1 tablespoon	31	0.0	0.00
Couscous, cooked	½ cup	100	0.1	0.03
Crab				
Blue, cooked	3 ounces	87	1.5	0.19
King, cooked	3 ounces	82	1.3	0.11
Crackers				
Butter	1 each	17	1.0	—
Graham, plain	1 square	30	0.5	—
Melba rounds, plain	1 each	11	0.2	—
Saltine	1 each	13	0.4	—
Cranberries				
Fresh, whole	½ cup	23	0.1	0.01
Juice cocktail, reduced-calorie	½ cup	22	0.0	0.00
Juice cocktail, regular	½ cup	75	0.1	0.00
Sauce, sweetened	¼ cup	105	0.1	0.01
Cream				
Half-and-half	1 tablespoon	20	1.7	1.08
Sour	1 tablespoon	31	3.0	1.88
Sour, nonfat	1 tablespoon	10	0.0	—
Sour, reduced-calorie	1 tablespoon	20	1.8	1.12
Whipping, unwhipped	1 tablespoon	51	5.5	3.43
Creamer, nondairy, powder	1 teaspoon	11	0.7	0.64
Croutons, seasoned	1 ounce	139	5.0	—
Cucumber, raw, whole	1 medium	32	0.3	0.08
Currants	1 tablespoon	25	0.0	0.00
Dates, pitted, unsweetened	5 each	114	0.2	0.08
Doughnut				
Cake-type	1 each	156	7.4	1.92
Plain, yeast	1 each	166	10.7	2.60
Egg				
White	1 each	16	0.0	0.00
Whole	1 each	77	5.2	1.61
Yolk	1 each	61	5.2	1.61
Substitute	¼ cup	30	0.0	0.00
Eggplant, cooked without salt	½ cup	13	0.1	0.02
Extract, vanilla	1 teaspoon	15	0.0	—
Fennel, leaves, raw	½ cup	13	0.2	—
Figs, dried	1 each	48	0.2	0.04
Fish, cooked				
Cod	3 ounces	89	0.7	0.14
Grouper	3 ounces	100	1.1	0.25
Halibut	3 ounces	119	2.5	0.35

FOOD	APPROXIMATE MEASURE	FOOD ENERGY (CALORIES)	FAT (GRAMS)	SATURATED FAT (GRAMS)
Fish *(continued)*				
Mackerel	3 ounces	134	5.4	1.53
Mahimahi	3 ounces	93	0.8	0.20
Perch	3 ounces	100	1.0	0.20
Pompano	3 ounces	179	10.3	3.83
Salmon, sockeye	3 ounces	184	9.3	1.63
Snapper	3 ounces	109	1.5	0.31
Sole	3 ounces	100	1.3	0.31
Swordfish	3 ounces	132	4.4	1.20
Tilapia	3 ounces	84	2.0	—
Trout	3 ounces	128	3.7	0.71
Tuna, canned in water, drained	3 ounces	111	0.4	0.14
Flour				
All-purpose, unsifted	1 cup	455	1.2	0.19
Bread, sifted	1 cup	495	2.3	0.33
Cake, sifted	1 cup	395	0.9	0.14
Whole wheat, unsifted	1 cup	407	2.2	0.39
Frankfurter				
All-meat	1 each	138	12.6	4.63
Chicken	1 each	113	8.6	—
Turkey	1 each	103	8.5	2.65
Fruit cocktail, canned, packed in juice	½ cup	57	0.0	0.00
Garlic, raw	1 clove	4	0.0	0.00
Gelatin				
Flavored, prepared with water	½ cup	81	0.0	—
Unflavored	1 teaspoon	10	0.0	—
Ginger				
Fresh, grated	1 teaspoon	1	0.0	0.00
Crystallized	1 ounce	96	0.1	—
Grapefruit				
Fresh	1 medium	77	0.2	0.03
Juice, unsweetened	½ cup	47	0.1	0.02
Grape juice, Concord	½ cup	60	0.0	—
Grapes, green, seedless	1 cup	114	0.9	0.30
Grits, cooked	½ cup	73	0.2	0.04
Ham				
Cured, roasted, extra-lean	3 ounces	123	4.7	1.54
Reduced-fat, low-salt	3 ounces	104	4.2	—
Honey	1 tablespoon	64	0.0	0.00
Honeydew, raw, diced	1 cup	59	0.2	0.08
Horseradish, prepared	1 tablespoon	6	0.0	0.01
Hot sauce, bottled	¼ teaspoon	0	0.0	—
Ice cream				
Chocolate, regular	½ cup	147	7.5	4.62
Chocolate, fat-free	½ cup	100	0.0	0.00
Vanilla, regular	½ cup	134	7.2	4.39
Vanilla, fat-free	½ cup	100	0.0	0.00
Jams and Jellies				
Regular	1 tablespoon	54	0.0	0.01
Reduced-calorie	1 tablespoon	29	0.0	—

FOOD	APPROXIMATE MEASURE	FOOD ENERGY (CALORIES)	FAT (GRAMS)	SATURATED FAT (GRAMS)
Jicama, diced	1 cup	49	0.2	0.07
Ketchup				
Regular	1 tablespoon	18	0.1	0.01
Reduced-calorie	1 tablespoon	7	0.0	—
Kiwifruit	1 each	44	0.5	0.08
Lamb				
Leg, roasted	3 ounces	162	6.6	2.35
Loin or chop, broiled	3 ounces	184	8.3	2.96
Rib, broiled	3 ounces	200	11.0	3.95
Lard	1 tablespoon	116	12.8	5.03
Leeks, sliced, raw	½ cup	32	0.2	0.03
Lemon				
Fresh	1 each	22	0.3	0.04
Juice	1 tablespoon	3	0.0	0.01
Lemonade, sweetened	1 cup	99	0.0	0.01
Lentils, cooked	½ cup	115	0.4	0.05
Lettuce				
Belgian endive	1 cup	14	0.1	0.02
Boston or Bibb, shredded	1 cup	7	0.1	0.02
Curly endive or escarole	1 cup	8	0.1	0.02
Iceberg, chopped	1 cup	7	0.1	0.01
Radicchio, raw	1 cup	10	0.1	—
Romaine, chopped	1 cup	9	0.1	0.01
Lime				
Fresh	1 each	20	0.1	0.01
Juice	1 tablespoon	4	0.0	0.00
Lobster, cooked, meat only	3 ounces	83	0.5	0.09
Mango, raw, cut into pieces	½ cup	54	0.2	0.05
Margarine				
Regular	1 tablespoon	101	11.4	2.23
Reduced-calorie, stick	1 tablespoon	50	5.6	0.93
Marshmallows, miniature	½ cup	73	0.0	0.00
Mayonnaise				
Regular	1 tablespoon	99	10.9	1.62
Nonfat	1 tablespoon	12	0.0	—
Reduced-calorie	1 tablespoon	44	4.6	0.70
Milk				
Buttermilk, nonfat	1 cup	88	0.8	0.64
Chocolate, low-fat, 1%	1 cup	158	2.5	1.55
Condensed, sweetened, low-fat	1 cup	960	12.0	8.0
Evaporated, skim, canned	1 cup	200	0.5	0.31
Low-fat, 1%	1 cup	102	2.5	1.61
Low-fat, 2%	1 cup	122	4.7	2.93
Nonfat dry	⅓ cup	145	0.3	0.20
Skim	1 cup	86	0.4	0.28
Whole	1 cup	149	8.1	5.05
Molasses, cane, light	1 tablespoon	52	0.0	—
Mushrooms				
Fresh	½ cup	9	0.1	0.02
Shiitake, dried	1 each	14	0.0	0.01
Mussels, blue, cooked	3 ounces	146	3.8	0.02

FOOD	APPROXIMATE MEASURE	FOOD ENERGY (CALORIES)	FAT (GRAMS)	SATURATED FAT (GRAMS)
Mustard				
Dijon	1 tablespoon	18	1.0	—
Prepared, yellow	1 tablespoon	12	0.7	0.03
Nectarine, fresh	1 each	67	0.6	0.07
Nuts				
Almonds, chopped	1 tablespoon	48	4.2	0.40
Hazelnuts, chopped	1 tablespoon	45	4.5	0.32
Macadamia, roasted, unsalted	1 tablespoon	60	6.4	0.96
Peanuts, roasted, unsalted	1 tablespoon	53	4.5	0.62
Pecans, chopped	1 tablespoon	50	5.0	0.40
Pine nuts	1 tablespoon	52	5.1	0.78
Pistachio nuts	1 tablespoon	46	3.9	0.49
Walnuts, black	1 tablespoon	47	4.4	0.28
Oats				
Cooked	1 cup	145	2.3	0.42
Rolled, dry	½ cup	156	2.6	0.45
Oil				
Canola	1 tablespoon	117	13.6	0.97
Corn	1 tablespoon	121	13.6	1.73
Olive	1 tablespoon	119	13.5	1.82
Sesame	1 tablespoon	121	13.6	1.92
Okra, cooked	½ cup	26	0.1	0.04
Olives				
Green, stuffed	1 medium	4	0.4	—
Ripe	1 medium	5	0.4	0.08
Onions				
Green, chopped	1 tablespoon	2	0.0	0.00
Raw, chopped	½ cup	32	0.1	0.02
Orange				
Fresh	1 medium	62	0.2	0.02
Juice	½ cup	56	0.1	0.01
Mandarin, canned, packed in juice	½ cup	46	0.0	0.00
Oysters, raw	3 ounces	59	2.1	0.54
Papaya				
Fresh, cubed	½ cup	27	0.1	0.03
Nectar, canned	½ cup	71	0.3	0.06
Parsley, raw	1 tablespoon	1	0.0	0.00
Parsnips, cooked, diced	½ cup	63	0.2	0.04
Passion fruit	1 medium	17	0.1	—
Pasta, cooked				
Macaroni or lasagna noodles	½ cup	99	0.5	0.07
Medium egg noodles	½ cup	106	1.2	0.25
Spaghetti or fettuccine	½ cup	99	0.5	0.07
Spinach noodles	½ cup	100	1.0	0.15
Whole wheat	½ cup	100	1.4	0.18
Peach				
Fresh	1 medium	37	0.1	0.01
Canned, packed in juice	½ cup	55	0.0	0.00
Juice	½ cup	57	0.0	—
Peanut butter				
Regular	1 tablespoon	95	8.3	1.38
Reduced-fat	1 tablespoon	90	6.0	1.00

FOOD	APPROXIMATE MEASURE	FOOD ENERGY (CALORIES)	FAT (GRAMS)	SATURATED FAT (GRAMS)
Pear				
Fresh	1 medium	97	0.7	0.03
Canned, packed in juice	½ cup	62	0.1	0.00
Peas				
Black-eyed, cooked	½ cup	90	0.7	0.17
English, cooked	½ cup	62	0.2	0.04
Snow pea pods, cooked or raw	½ cup	34	0.2	0.03
Split, cooked	½ cup	116	0.4	0.05
Sugar Snap, cooked or raw	½ cup	42	0.2	0.04
Peppers				
Chile, hot, green, chopped	1 tablespoon	4	0.0	0.00
Sweet, raw, green, red, or yellow	1 medium	19	0.4	0.05
Phyllo pastry, raw	1 sheet	57	1.1	0.17
Pickle				
Dill, sliced	¼ cup	4	0.1	0.02
Relish, chopped, sour	1 tablespoon	3	0.1	—
Sweet, sliced	¼ cup	57	0.2	0.04
Pie, baked, 9-inch diameter, cut into 8 slices				
Apple	1 slice	409	15.3	5.22
Chocolate meringue	1 slice	354	13.4	5.38
Peach	1 slice	327	11.0	2.74
Pecan	1 slice	478	20.3	4.31
Pimiento, diced	1 tablespoon	4	0.1	0.01
Pineapple				
Fresh, diced	½ cup	38	0.3	0.02
Canned, packed in juice	½ cup	75	0.1	0.01
Juice, unsweetened	½ cup	70	0.1	0.01
Plum, fresh	1 medium	35	0.4	0.03
Popcorn, hot-air popped	1 cup	23	0.3	0.04
Pork, cooked				
Chop, center-loin	3 ounces	204	11.1	—
Tenderloin	3 ounces	141	4.1	1.41
Potato				
Baked, with skin	1 each	218	0.2	0.05
Boiled, diced	½ cup	67	0.1	0.02
Potato chips	10 each	105	7.1	1.81
Pretzel sticks, thin	10 each	25	0.5	—
Prunes				
Dried, pitted	1 each	20	0.0	0.00
Juice	½ cup	91	0.0	0.00
Pumpkin, canned	½ cup	42	0.3	0.18
Radish, fresh, sliced	½ cup	10	0.3	0.01
Raisins	1 tablespoon	27	0.0	0.01
Raspberries, red, fresh	½ cup	30	0.3	0.01
Rhubarb				
Raw, diced	½ cup	13	0.1	0.02
Cooked, with sugar	½ cup	157	0.1	0.01
Rice, cooked without salt or fat				
Brown	½ cup	110	0.9	—
White, long-grain	½ cup	108	0.1	—
Wild	½ cup	83	0.3	0.04

FOOD	APPROXIMATE MEASURE	FOOD ENERGY (CALORIES)	FAT (GRAMS)	SATURATED FAT (GRAMS)
Rice cake, plain	1 each	36	0.2	0.00
Roll				
Croissant	1 each	272	17.3	10.67
Hard	1 each	156	1.6	0.35
Kaiser, small	1 each	92	1.8	—
Plain, brown-and-serve	1 each	82	2.0	0.34
Rutabaga, cooked, cubed	½ cup	29	0.2	0.02
Salad dressing				
Blue cheese, low-calorie	1 tablespoon	59	5.8	1.40
Cucumber, fat-free, creamy	1 tablespoon	8	0.0	0.00
French, low-calorie	1 tablespoon	20	0.0	0.00
Italian, no-oil, low-calorie	1 tablespoon	8	0.0	—
Ranch-style, fat-free	1 tablespoon	16	0.0	0.00
Thousand Island, low-calorie	1 tablespoon	24	1.6	0.25
Salsa, commercial	1 tablespoon	3	0.0	—
Salt, iodized	1 teaspoon	0	0.0	0.00
Sauces				
Barbecue	2 tablespoons	23	0.5	—
Tartar, regular	2 tablespoons	143	15.2	2.35
Sauerkraut, canned	½ cup	22	0.2	0.04
Scallops, raw, large	3 ounces	75	0.6	0.07
Sesame seeds, dry, whole	1 teaspoon	17	1.5	0.21
Sherbet				
Lime or raspberry	½ cup	104	0.9	—
Orange	½ cup	135	1.9	1.19
Shortening	1 tablespoon	113	12.6	2.36
Shrimp, cooked, peeled, and deveined	3 ounces	84	0.9	0.25
Soup, condensed, made with water				
Chicken noodle	1 cup	75	2.4	0.65
Chili, beef	1 cup	170	6.6	—
Cream of chicken, low-salt, reduced-fat	1 cup	80	2.5	1.00
Cream of mushroom, low-salt, reduced-fat	1 cup	70	3.0	1.00
Cream of potato	1 cup	73	2.3	1.22
Onion	1 cup	58	1.7	—
Tomato	1 cup	85	1.9	0.37
Vegetable, beef	1 cup	78	2.0	0.83
Soy sauce				
Regular	1 tablespoon	8	0.0	0.00
Low-sodium	1 tablespoon	6	0.0	0.00
Spinach				
Fresh	1 cup	12	0.2	0.03
Cooked	½ cup	21	0.2	0.04
Squash, cooked				
Acorn	½ cup	57	0.1	0.03
Butternut	½ cup	41	0.1	0.02
Spaghetti	½ cup	22	0.2	0.05
Summer	½ cup	18	0.3	0.06
Strawberries, fresh	1 cup	45	0.6	0.03
Sugar				
Granulated	1 tablespoon	48	0.0	0.00
Brown, packed	1 tablespoon	51	0.0	—
Powdered	1 tablespoon	29	0.0	0.00

FOOD	APPROXIMATE MEASURE	FOOD ENERGY (CALORIES)	FAT (GRAMS)	SATURATED FAT (GRAMS)
Sweet potato				
Whole, baked	1 each	103	0.1	0.02
Mashed	½ cup	172	0.5	0.10
Syrup				
Chocolate-flavored	1 tablespoon	49	0.2	0.00
Corn, dark or light	1 tablespoon	60	0.0	0.00
Maple, reduced-calorie	1 tablespoon	30	0.2	0.00
Pancake	1 tablespoon	50	0.0	0.00
Taco shell	1 each	52	2.8	—
Tangerine, fresh	1 medium	38	0.1	0.02
Tapioca, dry	1 tablespoon	32	0.0	—
Tofu, firm	4 ounces	164	9.9	1.43
Tomato				
Fresh	1 medium	26	0.4	0.06
Dried	1 ounce	73	0.8	0.12
Dried, packed in oil	1 ounce	60	4.0	0.54
Juice, no-salt-added	1 cup	41	0.1	0.02
Paste, no-salt-added	1 tablespoon	11	0.0	—
Sauce, no-salt-added	½ cup	40	0.0	—
Whole, canned, no-salt-added	½ cup	22	0.0	—
Tortilla				
Corn, 6-inch diameter	1 each	67	1.1	0.12
Flour, 6-inch diameter	1 each	111	2.3	0.56
Turkey, skinned, boned, and roasted				
White meat	3 ounces	134	2.7	0.87
Dark meat	3 ounces	159	6.1	2.06
Sausage link or patty	1 ounce	55	3.2	1.00
Turnip greens, cooked	½ cup	14	0.2	0.04
Turnips, cooked, cubed	½ cup	14	0.1	0.01
Veal, cooked				
Leg	3 ounces	128	2.9	1.04
Loin	3 ounces	149	5.9	2.19
Vegetable juice cocktail, low-sodium	1 cup	48	0.2	—
Vinegar, distilled	1 tablespoon	2	0.0	0.00
Water chestnuts, canned, sliced	½ cup	35	0.0	0.01
Watermelon, diced	1 cup	51	0.7	0.35
Wheat germ	1 tablespoon	26	0.7	0.12
Whipped cream	1 tablespoon	26	2.8	1.71
Whipped topping, nondairy frozen	1 tablespoon	15	1.2	1.02
Wonton wrapper	1 each	6	0.1	0.03
Worcestershire sauce, low-sodium	1 tablespoon	12	0.0	0.00
Yeast, active, dry	1 package	20	0.1	0.01
Yogurt				
Coffee and vanilla, low-fat	1 cup	193	2.8	1.84
Frozen, nonfat	½ cup	82	0.0	0.00
Fruit varieties, low-fat	1 cup	225	2.6	1.68
Plain, nonfat	1 cup	127	0.4	0.26
Zucchini, cooked, diced	½ cup	17	0.1	0.01

INDEX